Into the Jaws of Yama, Lord of Death

Into the Jaws of Yama, Lord of Death

Buddhism, Bioethics and Death

KARMA LEKSHE TSOMO

STATE UNIVERSITY OF NEW YORK PRESS

Graphic design of Yama image courtesy of Daphne Chu and Michel Le, Ostrander & Chu.

Published by
State University of New York Press, Albany

For information, address State University of New York Press,
194 Washington Avenue, Suite 305, Albany, NY 12210-2384

Production by Kelli Williams
Marketing by Susan M. Petrie

Library of Congress Cataloging-in-Publication Data

Karma Lekshe Tsomo, 1944–
  Into the jaws of Yama, lord of death : Buddhism, bioethics, and death / Karma Lekshe Tsomo.
    p. cm.
  Includes bibliographical references and index.
  ISBN-13: 978-0-7914-6831-9 (hardcover : alk. paper)
  ISBN-10: 0-7914-6831-3 (hardcover : alk. paper)
  ISBN-13: 978-0-7914-6832-6 (pbk. : alk. paper)
  ISBN-10: 0-7914-6832-1 (pbk. : alk. paper)
  1. Death—Religious aspects—Buddhism. 2. Intermediate state—Buddhism.
3. Buddhism—Doctrines. I. Title.

BQ4487.K375 2006
294.3'5697—dc22   2005030347

10 9 8 7 6 5 4 3 2 1

This book is dedicated to my parents,
who taught me about life and death.
Martha Jean Haycraft Walters
1918–2001
and
Philip Zenn
1919–2005

Contents

Acknowledgments

This study draws on the insights of numerous scholars and friends, gleaned through readings and discussions over many years. For their friendship, editorial skills, and wisdom, I would like to express my heartfelt appreciation to Ramona Bajema, Margaret Coberly, Evelyn Diane Cowie, Ahna Fender, and Rebecca Paxton. For his unfailing patience and compassion, I am especially indebted to my mentor and friend David W. Chappel (1940–2004). For their continual guidance and encouragement during an overextended university career, I am also most grateful to University of Hawaiʻi, Mānoa, professors Eliot Deutsch, Roger Ames, Arindam Chakrabarti, Graham Parkes, and Samuel Shapiro. For the grants and scholarships that helped sustain me during the initial stages of the research, I acknowledge with appreciation the East-West Center, the Buddhist Studies Program and Center for South Asian Studies of the University of Hawaiʻi School of Hawaiian, Asian, and Pacific Studies, Fakuang Institute, Rocky Foundation, and Zenkoji Scholarship Foundation. For the institutional support and warm collegiality that have allowed me to complete the final manuscript, I am deeply grateful to my associates at the University of San Diego. For their illuminating commentaries on these texts and teachings, I am profoundly grateful to His Holiness the Fourteenth Dalai Lama, Geshe Ngawang Dhargyey, Geshe Rapten, Geshe Damchö Gyaltsen, Geshe Sonam Rinchen, and Kalu Rinpoche. All errors are entirely my own.

Chapter 1

Introduction

As a small child, I was fascinated with the question of what happens after death. An aura of mystery, fear, and avoidance seemed to accompany the topic of death. Although I asked one authority after another, the answers did not strike me as satisfactory. The rewards of heaven and the threat of hell did not seem convincing explanations of what happens to human beings after the breath stops and the eyes close. I continued to search, ultimately looking further afield to find an answer to this puzzle. My search led me to many countries in Asia and eventually to the Tibetan refugee settlement of Dharamsala in northern India.

After my third serious bout of hepatitis during my studies in Dharamsala, I naïvely asked a Tibetan doctor, "Am I going to die?" Dr. Yeshi Dhonden, the private physician to His Holiness the Dalai Lama, immediately replied, "Of course, you're going to die! We're all going to die!" Clearly, his personal perspective on life and death was intimately in tune with the descriptions of death and dying I had been studying in Tibetan Buddhist texts.

Some years later, as I lay for three months in hospitals in Delhi and Tijuana recovering from a poisonous viper bite, the prospect of death loomed very near. The medical staff in Delhi did not expect me to survive and for several weeks after receiving the poisonous bite, I dwelled in a liminal realm between consciousness and unconsciousness that bore little resemblance to ordinary waking reality. Every day death was imminent, particularly in view of the medical care available. After one particular surgery, the staff saw me turn blue and I awakened in what appeared to be another realm of existence. As I was wheeled out of the operating theater, through a blue haze, three

1

unknown Indian blood donors standing at the foot of the bed appeared to be angels. The experience of living on the edge of death for so long rekindled the questions about death that had fascinated me as a child.

In 1995, the University of Hawai'i at Mānoa School of Hawaiian, Asian, and Pacific Studies (SHAPS) sponsored a six-week project on Living and Dying in Buddhist Cultures, both as a summer session course and as a community outreach effort. The six-week program focused on attitudes toward death and dying in a variety of different cultures: Hawaiian, Chinese, Japanese, Korean, Thai, Tibetan, and Vietnamese. In the process of directing this project, I became fascinated by the multiplicity of approaches to dying. As I edited the proceedings for a handbook of Buddhist approaches to dying and a series of video programs, many questions arose that challenged traditional Eurocentric notions of death and the afterlife. Gradually I began to realize that gaining a cross-cultural understanding of attitudes toward death and dying has real practical value. It is valuable not only for health care professionals, who deal with questions of life and death on a daily basis, but also for educators, social workers, caregivers, and the general public. Especially in view of new medical technologies, and in today's increasingly multicultural society, it is essential to develop an understanding of different cultural attitudes toward death.

In the course of preparing this manuscript, both of my parents passed away. Suddenly and in a very personal way, I was confronted with the very questions I had been researching academically. Quickly it became obvious that losing a close loved one is an entirely different experience than developing a theoretical analysis about the topic of death. Not only is it a more immediate and emotional experience, but many more factors affect coping, understanding, and decision making than meet the scholarly eye. From these experiences, I learned more than any book could teach me about the questions that need to be asked and the resources available to help make wise and compassionate decisions about end-of-life care.

Toward New Understandings of Death

Death is perhaps the most urgent topic of all philosophical speculation, yet it is a topic we tend to avoid since it threatens our very existence and challenges our assumptions about an eternal, solid self. Sophisticated modern societies have become especially adept at denying death and hiding it behind a facade of youth, vitality, and beauty. At one point, it seemed that death had replaced sex as a social taboo.

In recent years, however, the nuclear and biological dangers that threaten life and the advances in medical technology that prolong life have made a reexamination of death imperative. Death will inevitably come to all living beings, and therefore holds great significance for the living. Death is a paradox, because it is both a personal concern and a social concern. It is especially painful because when a loved one dies, the personal realm and the external social spheres collide, such that our innermost feelings frequently become the object of public scrutiny. Death is a further paradox because it is at once universal and culture-specific. It is for this reason that cross-cultural perspectives on death hold the potential to enrich our common human understanding.

But what is death, and what is it that dies? From a Buddhist perspective, personal identity is constructed in dependence on various physical and psychological components and death is the dissolution of those components. If death were merely the disintegration of the physical body, human beings should feel no greater sadness at a person's death than they feel at the loss of any other material item. The fact that the death of a human being or an animal can cause a far greater sense of loss than the loss of a material thing raises important questions about the psychological components of personal identity and what becomes of them at the time of death.

Questions about death and personal identity have been integral to Buddhist thought for over twenty-five hundred years. The way in which these questions have been addressed by scholars and practitioners in Buddhist cultures suggests new directions for inquiry that may be especially useful in a consideration of ethical dilemmas. Many of the bioethical questions raised by new medical technologies remain unresolved, and religion is often seen as interfering with law and medicine. A consideration of these unresolved controversies requires open-minded inquiry, from every possible vantage point. An examination of Buddhist ideas on these topics is not only a convenient focus for understanding various Buddhist philosophical perspectives and cultures, but it may also open new lines of inquiry in Western thought.

Recent public debates on abortion, for example, have raised questions about the sanctity of human life, the status of a fetus as a full conscious being, the ethics of surrogacy, and a woman's rights over her own body. Debates on euthanasia, assisted suicide, and organ transplantation similarly raise questions about moral agency, quality of life, the ethics of extending life, and the rights of human beings to terminate their own lives. Because death is such a central focus of Buddhist philosophy, it has stimulated centuries of inquiry and analysis that may be useful in the current debates. Buddhist

approaches to these questions, based as they are on a specific set of
assumptions about death, personhood, and moral agency, introduce
new ways of thinking about these highly controversial issues. Utilizing the framework of Buddhist philosophy may contribute insights
that will spark new directions and ways of thinking about a continually expanding range of bioethical issues.

The Face of Death

When one enters a Buddhist retreat center in Thailand, it is not un-
common to be greeted by a full human skeleton suspended from the
top of its frame, a grim reminder of the inevitable outcome of life.
Similarly, when one enters a Tibetan retreat center or monastery, one
is likely to be met by a painting of the wheel of becoming. The wheel
is divided in concentric circles: the outer circle depicts the twelve links
of dependent arising, beginning with ignorance, that explain how
sentient beings become entangled in the dismal cycle of birth and
death (saṃsāra). The middle circle depicts the six realms of rebirth into
which sentient beings may be born after death. The central circle depicts a rooster, snake, and pig, representing the three mental defilements of greed, hatred, and ignorance that keep beings spinning from
one rebirth to the next. Above the wheel Yama, the Lord of Death,
drools in anticipation of his victims. The wheel of becoming as a whole
represents saṃsāra, the vicious cycle of existence in which ordinary
beings are trapped.

The skeletons and images of dying found in Buddhist monasteries remind us that death is inevitable for all living beings. Among the
more than six billion people currently inhabiting the Earth, all face
the same inescapable end. Regardless of race, class, or gender, death
is the most fundamental human experience. One of the most basic,
defining aspects of a culture is the way it responds to death. What
fresh perspectives do the Buddhist philosophical traditions bring to a
discussion of our common human destiny?

Most Buddhist adherents view death as a wake-up call, a reminder of impermanence and the preciousness of human life. Despite
the infinite expanse of time and notions of personal continuity assumed by early Indian religious and philosophical traditions, the duration of a specific lifetime is brief and uncertain. From the moment of
birth, our lives flow inescapably toward death. For Buddhists, this
inevitability inveighs against frivolity and mediocrity, and prompts
the thoughtful to weigh their priorities against some higher standard
of value.

Although death is unavoidable, the conditions of its occurrence often invite moral judgment. Suicides, drug casualties, deaths from self-destructive behavior, and capital punishment, for example, are deemed blameworthy, denounced as "wasted lives" or "just deserts." Other cases, condemned by circumstances, are labeled "a bad death," "an unworthy death," "a tragic death," or "an untimely death." Still other deaths may be commended, as in "good," "honorable," or "courageous" deaths. Death may be viewed as a moral imperative, such as Arjuna's mandate to avenge his kinsfolk in the *Bhagavadgītā* or the custom of *satī*, a woman's immolation on her husband's funeral pyre. Death may be a social or personal imperative, as when a Japanese executive commits suicide to atone for his own or his company's negligence; a national imperative, as a patriotic duty in war; or a medical imperative, as in some cases of euthanasia or assisted suicide. Even the most innocuous death may be judged "sad" or "premature."

Some construe death as the final measure of a person's life. Whether death is viewed as the completion of a life well-lived, the welcome conclusion of a painful illness, or simply the terminus of one's present worldly experience, death is undeniably the extinction of one individual's current possibilities. In many cultural narratives, including the varied Buddhist narratives, the positive and negative deeds of a lifetime are weighed to determine a person's destiny. This prevalent cultural motif is consistent with the life review often reported after near-death experiences. Death as the measure of one's life is illustrated literally in the Chinese hell scrolls, where a judge resembling a Confucian bureaucrat calculates the account balance of one's virtues and vices. Parallel images are drawn in Buddhist literature, where white and black stones symbolizing wholesome and unwholesome deeds are weighed by Māra, the Evil One, "the god of lust, sin, and death." For Buddhists, death is a moment of reckoning—epitomizing the thoughts and actions of our lifetime and determining our future after death. Death is not just a singular event, but a process of transition, whether to awakening or future rebirth.

Why Death is Important

Paradoxically, although death is the end of all life's achievements and pleasures, it also serves as a catalyst for understanding life's ultimate value. Why does death acquire such importance and how does the finality of death affect the way we live our lives? How can human beings meaningfully prepare for death when they have no firsthand knowledge of it? What about death is culturally specific and what is universal to all living beings, bridging cultural differences? How do our understandings of death and personal identity inform the ethical choices we make?

Even though death is an uncomfortable topic, it continues to capture the human imagination. Deny or ignore death as we may, it is all around us—in the morning news, in the falling leaves, in the falling of our hair, and in countless other reminders. The recent global AIDS epidemic has forced the complicated, often frightening issues around dying to the foreground of public awareness. Films on death and rebirth appear one after the other, not to mention thousands of films involving murder. What makes death so intriguing?

Death is, beyond dispute, a universal terminus for all living beings, yet paradoxically it is an experience about which the living have no firsthand information. The threat of death looms for the living, but it is not clear why death presents such a threat. When death looms, it has the effect of accentuating our relationships and our understanding of life. Yet when death arrives, everything that has been most dear to us, including our carefully crafted identity with its memories, opinions, and preferences, becomes totally irrelevant.

Life Beyond Death: A Persistent Claim

The contention that human beings are solely material entities of flesh, bone, liquid, and air has major implications for how we live our lives and how we die. If there is no soul or afterlife, then death is simply the end of a biological and psychological process—the inverse of life and a simple negative. The view that living beings' physical components are recycled may be some consolation, but does not satisfy the human mind's quest for meaning. While it may be true that death is as valuable as life itself, that notion may not give us much solace at the death of a loved one, or in facing our own death.

Death has different implications for a person who believes in the existence of a soul and one who does not, but the differences are not simple. The notion of a soul is generally couched in a religious belief system, often one that entails a supreme being, judgments, concepts of retribution and reward, and entitlements for believers. Despite the inroads of secularism, the belief in an afterlife still has a strong following. According to a 1996 survey by *Newsweek*, 96 percent of American people believe in heaven and 75 percent of them believe that they are going there; only 26 percent believe in hell and only 3 percent of them believe that they are going there. Although most people today seem to be more concerned with this life than the next, a belief in heaven and hell persists, with heaven definitely the more attractive option.

As is widely recognized, concepts of personal identity and ethics are constructed in early childhood, conditioned by family, education, society, and culture. In a number of human cultures, assumptions about past and future lives are part of this conditioning. Individual propensities, aptitudes, and affinities may be explained as the result of past life experiences. An individual is regarded as a composite of predispositions from past lives and the influences of environment, education, and life circumstances, as well as the individual's responses to these influences. This process of identity formation is exceedingly complex, complicated further by the physiological aspects of human development.

If death is simply a physiological event and there is nothing beyond death, then death wipes clean the slate of human virtues and transgressions. But there are moral and logical problems integral to this view. First, if death obliterates the traces of our actions, what is the motivating force for ethical living? If actions have no effects beyond this life, what prevents humanity from deteriorating into chaos and evil? Second, even if it is impossible to substantiate rebirth, is it possible to disprove it? The fact that human beings do not remember past lives is not sufficient evidence to prove that they do not exist. Remembrances of past lives have been documented, and if past lives exist, it is possible that future lives exist as well. In many cultures the possibility of rebirth seems at least as likely as the spontaneous occurrence of sentient life without cause. In Buddhist cultures, it is believed that rebirth can be verified through direct perception by skilled yogis, as a by-product of intensive meditation practice, and that this knowledge is therefore theoretically accessible. In the absence of conclusive proof to the contrary, even many ordinary people accept the possibility that their actions may produce results beyond this life, just as actions within an individual lifetime have consequences.

Death and Rebirth Across Cultures

Although the idea of other lives may be discounted or viewed as simply an expedient to allay fears of death, it is a common aspect of many world cultures, both Asian and Western. In *Meno*, Plato speaks of an immortal soul that gains knowledge and experience through an endless round of deaths and rebirths: "Thus the soul, since it is immortal and has been born many times, and has seen all things both here and in the other world, has learned everything that is."[1] This perspective coincides with that of Empedocles, who recalls: "For already have I once been a boy and a girl, a fish and a bird and a dumb sea fish."[2] In the *Republic*, drawing on the after-death experience of a Pamphylian named Er, Plato speaks of a literal judgment of souls similar to that portrayed in Chinese hell scrolls. He speaks of heavenly rewards for good deeds and dreadful punishments for bad deeds, including a tenfold escalation of retribution analogous to the exponential increase in karmic consequences described in Buddhist texts.

Buddhist ruminations on death have further counterparts in Greek philosophy. Socrates, for example, characterized philosophy as "practicing dying." This mirrors the standard Buddhist practice of rehearsing one's own dying. This practice may be viewed as dying to the world prematurely, dissociating from the body to evade death's sting, or artificially depriving oneself of life's full enjoyment. But, for Buddhists, life's pleasures are ephemeral and largely deceptive; this short lifetime will be over all too soon, and attachment to the pleasures of the world only makes dying that much more difficult. Through rehearsing the experience of dying, a practitioner is more likely to live with heightened awareness and appreciation, referred to in Zen as "living having let go of life." An awareness of the imminence of death imbues life with greater intensity and meaning.

A notion of personal identity that extends beyond death was also common among the ancient Greeks. The Orphics believed in the transmigration of souls; they had specific instructions designed to guide them through the perils of the next world and to "escape from the wheel of birth." Pythagoras believed that the body entombs the soul and that things are born again and again in a cyclical pattern. Possibly influenced by Indian thought, he believed that the soul is capable of transformation and release from the wheel of repeated rebirth.

Constructions of Personal Identity: What Dies?

Buddhist texts and teachers frequently state that living beings hold nothing so dear as their own lives. Understanding the nature of the self has been a central topic of Buddhist inquiry from the start because the self is the locus of a person's experience. All experiences, whether pleasant, unpleasant, or neutral, are experienced by oneself. And, according to the Buddhists, whether one experiences happiness or misery is a result of one's own actions and perceptions. But, for Buddhists, the self is merely a label given to a set of components. The belief in an independently existent self is a mistaken perception with serious consequences, for all afflictions are rooted in a fundamental misconception about the nature of the self. Grasping at the mistaken perceptions of oneself and other phenomena leads to constant frustrations, anxieties, and unhappiness. Understanding the illusory nature of the self allows one to experience things "as they are," without interference from conceptual constructs.

In the Buddhist view, grasping at a mistaken view of the self and the world is the source of profound disillusionment. All afflictions arise from identifying with a false sense of self, whereas great contentment arises from seeing the true nature of things. If one believes that the self exists solidly and independently, as it appears, then the dissolution of the self at death is a disaster. But if the self is understood to be illusory from the beginning, the dissolution of the self at death is simply another opportunity for awakening. The conventional self is simply a convenient designation for the everyday collection of transitory aggregates: body, feelings, recognitions, karmic formations, and consciousness. Ultimately, the self as a permanent entity is an illusion and all attempts to elevate the self merely compound the illusion. The stronger one grasps at the illusory self, the more one suffers when the illusion shatters.

Persons as Moral Agents

Constructions of personal identity are integral to personal and social ethics, especially in matters of bioethics. Patterns of ethical decision making reflect differences in family structures and these patterns change as family structures change. For example, individuals who are raised to be independent decision makers may view end-of-life decisions as matters of personal choice, whereas individuals raised in close-knit families may approach these matters cooperatively, as decisions affecting the whole family. New technologies are dramatically affecting opinions on life and death issues such as surrogate parenting, organ transplantation, physician-assisted suicide, and genetic engineering. The public uproar and legal wrangling over terminating artificial life support, as in the case of Terri Schiavo, reveal that advances in medical technologies have outstripped society's ability to neatly determine what is moral and what is not. The debate exposes deep fissures in the process of moral judgment that are both emotionally and politically charged.

Ethical decision making is influenced not only by cultural attitudes, but also by taboos and proscriptive regulations created and enforced through individual and group approval and censure. In their pivotal study on the interrelationship between cultural constructions of self and emotions, Hazel Rose Markus and Shinobu Kitayama demonstrated that actions, moral judgments, and decisions are made by a culturally constructed self in relation to culturally and socially defined values.[3] Understanding how culture affects individuals as moral agents helps us understand the values that influence human beings' bioethical decision making.

The aim here is to analyze the concepts of death and personal identity as they are understood in Buddhist metaphysics and to investigate what becomes of personal identity at the time of death. In the Buddhist view, there is no fixed concept of self; instead, there is a sequence of impermanent, dependently arising moments of consciousness. If the self is contingent and has no ontological status, however, this raises questions about how to develop a viable theory of moral agency and moral efficacy. If individuals have no true, independent existence, the Buddhists are pressed to explain how human beings generate delusions, create actions, experience joys and afflictions, and sow the seeds for future rebirths. These questions are not only problematic for Buddhists; the link between the individual and moral agency is an age-old conundrum.

Until recently, discussions about biomedical ethics have been based on theories of self and moral agency that have developed within a Western context. The primary goal of this book is to expand the conversation by exploring the issues of death, identity, and bioethics within a Buddhist framework, focusing especially on Tibet. Because all Buddhist traditions trace their roots to India, an exploration of Indian Buddhist views on death and personhood serves as a foundation for tracing further Buddhist philosophical developments. The earliest strata of Indian Buddhist texts describe the self as a label used to denote the conventionally existent person, based on five categories of momentary aggregates. The contingent, momentary nature of the self raises questions about moral agency, karma, and the continuity of consciousness after death. An exploration of these basic questions is crucial for understanding attitudes toward death in Buddhist cultures and for discussing such issues as suicide, abortion, and euthanasia. After discussing the philosophical foundations of Buddhist ethics in India, I focus on how these ideas were interpreted in Tibet and other Buddhist cultures. An understanding of the questions about death that have been the focus of so much philosophical inquiry among diverse Buddhist traditions over many generations will provide points of departure for discussing death in a multicultural context. These topics of inquiry will also provide a foundation for cross-cultural discussions about ethical values, dying with dignity, and end-of-life care.

The ephemeral nature of life, the inevitability of death, and the shifting nature of individual identity have all been acknowledged in

Buddhist cultures for centuries. For a very long time Buddhists and non-Buddhists in India debated the nature of the self, the workings of karma, and the continuity of consciousness. If self and consciousness are no more than contingent, momentary realities, then how are the impressions of positive and negative actions transmitted from one lifetime to the next? If there is no ultimately existing person, then who experiences the results of action? A satisfactory explanation for the paradoxical relationship between the doctrines of karma and selfless-ness is critical for establishing Buddhist ethics as a convincing frame-work for discussing present-day biomedical realities.

Tracing the Sources of Buddhist Ideas

The close encounters with dying that opened this chapter evoke a host of questions about the universal experience of death. The theories of consciousness, death, and rebirth that are discussed in early Indian Buddhist texts serve as a foundation not only for understanding sub-sequent Buddhist philosophical developments in Tibet and other Bud-dhist cultures, but also for understanding our own attitudes toward death and the possibility of an afterlife. The discussion of Buddhist views of death and how they were interpreted over time requires a grounding in Indian Buddhist viewpoints on the topic and a compara-tive analysis of Madhyamaka and Yogācāra, the two major streams of Mahāyāna Buddhist thought. These philosophical systems provide a framework for understanding death through Buddhist eyes.

The *Visuddhimagga*, written by Buddhaghoṣa in Pāli in the fifth century CE on the basis of Sinhalese commentaries, is important because it has become the standard interpretation of Buddhist doc-trine in the Theravāda tradition on the issues of self, rebirth, and personal continuity. Vasubandhu's commentary on the *Abhidharmakośa* is equally significant because it presents a Mahāyāna viewpoint from a subsequent time period and because it specifically addresses the theories of *karma*, rebirth, and the intermediate state. Dharmakīrti's *Pramāṇavārttikakārikā* provides a lucid analysis of the notion of self. The *Lamrim* texts, *Bardo Tödrol*, and other Tibetan texts are valuable resources for an understanding of Tibetan Buddhist views, especially on the nature of consciousness and the transference of consciousness at the time of death.

Buddhist understandings of death, personal identity, and rebirth all trace back to India, but they did not develop in a vacuum. As Buddhism spread to new lands and peoples, these understandings were informed by indigenous attitudes that predate the introduction of Buddhism. The process of diffusion and the subsequent intermingling of ideas and practices accounts for the different voices and the rich panoply of beliefs and customs related to death that we find in various Buddhist cultures. To understand the Buddhist attitudes and practices that differ from culture to culture, I examine the Indian Buddhist philosophical foundations of belief and praxis, and how they developed over time. To begin, I focus on several fundamental topics: the nature of death, the nature of consciousness, the apparent contradiction between the concepts of no-self (*anātman*) and rebirth, and the nature of personhood in the intermediate state (*antarābhāva*, Tibetan: *bardo*). Specific examples illustrate how these concepts were interpreted differently in Buddhist cultures. For example, when Buddhism entered Tibet in the seventh century, it was understood against a background of indigenous Bön beliefs and ritual practices. In this cultural environment, Tibetan scholars and practitioners developed unique practices related to death, using the experience of dying and the intermediate state between death and rebirth (*bardo*) as an opportunity for psychological transformation. In similar ways, Buddhist ideas were adopted and recast in other cultural milieu.

These topics lead naturally to a discussion of the ethical implications of the *anātman* theory for end-of-life decision making. To begin, I consider traditional formulations of Buddhist ethics and how these theories are related to questions about death and rebirth. Although Buddhist texts provide clear guidelines on some basic moral questions, such as abortion and suicide, they do not provide ready answers for the ethical complexities of the twenty-first century. The complicated issues raised by new medical technologies require a thorough understanding of Buddhist ethics and philosophy as a basis for thinking about the ethical implications of a whole new range of complex issues, such as organ transplantation, stem cell research, and cloning. To discuss these issues intelligently requires a familiarity with a whole new vocabulary, for example, the distinctions between suicide, assisted suicide, and euthanasia, and between the qualifiers voluntary and involuntary, active and passive. Further, it requires a recognition that specific philosophical and cultural premises underlie much of the dialogue on these issues to date. Expanding the conversation requires recognizing that these assumptions may or may not apply in other cultural contexts. It is therefore a timely opportunity to reexamine these assumptions. Buddhist attitudes about death and personal identity provide a different theoretical framework and new perspectives on end-of-life issues that can enrich contemporary discussions of bioethical issues.

The questions that Buddhism asks about life and death are questions that concern all thoughtful human beings. The accumulated wisdom of the Buddhist traditions shed light on what human beings can learn from these universal experiences. Whereas some aspects of Buddhist belief and practice attract attention because they appear unusual or exotic, other aspects attract attention because they deal with ordinary human emotions and experiences. Buddhists are being called upon to reflect on ancient Buddhist texts and traditions and how they are relevant to the challenges of society, technology, and politics today. Traditional Buddhist ethical ideals have stood the test of time in Asian societies, but now they are being tested in light of new realities unimaginable in the Buddha's day. If the Buddhist teachings have lasting value, then they must be applicable to the critical needs of the contemporary world. The rich variety of Buddhist philosophies and practices demonstrates the adaptability that has served the tradition well over many centuries, while at the same time maintaining the compassionate, nonviolent, tolerant core values that have made the tradition a source of hope and meaning for millions of people for ages. The willingness to engage with vastly different ideas and ways of living is a major asset in a world beset by violence, exploitation, and misunderstandings. The Buddha's agenda of creating human happiness seems more relevant than ever.

The objective of this analysis is not only an understanding of Buddhist attitudes toward death. Because death is a universal experience, an exploration of Buddhist approaches to death, personhood, and bioethics will also hopefully contribute to contemporary dialogue on these issues and take the conversation in new directions. Recent advances in biomedical technology have stimulated a surge of interest in death and bioethical issues such as abortion, cloning, euthanasia, organ transplantation, assisted suicide, and stem cell research. As the human life span lengthens and the time between the onset of old age and the final moment of death increases, these issues take on renewed urgency. Ethicists, health care providers, and ordinary individuals have begun to refine their questions, expand their awareness, and consider alternative ways of looking at a vast new array of issues.

A consideration of Buddhist theories unmasks certain assumptions inherent in the usual ways these issues and questions are framed in Western cultures. In the following chapters, I explore how a Buddhist analysis of these questions may open up lines of philosophical inquiry that will have practical relevance for social workers, hospice workers, health care professionals, and caregivers in today's increasingly multicultural communities. The questions raised and the diverse

Buddhist perspectives presented bring new voices to the conversations that are shaping legislation and public policy on what are likely to be some of the most controversial issues of the twenty-first century.

Chapter 2

Understanding Death and Impermanence

One day in June 1963, Thich Quang Duc, a highly respected Vietnamese Buddhist monk, sat outside the Cambodian Embassy on a noisy thoroughfare in Saigon to protest the oppression of Buddhists by the United States-backed regime of the Catholic dictator Ngo Dinh Diem. Dressed in traditional orange Buddhist robes and surrounded by a chanting circle of devoted supporters, the monk quietly doused himself with petrol and, seated in the lotus position, was soon engulfed in flames. This powerful image of a Buddhist monk's self-immolation is deeply ingrained in the historical consciousness of American social activists, the Vietnamese people, and ordinary television viewers around the world. His action, often cited as a turning point in toppling Diem's corrupt and autocratic regime, eventually led to the withdrawal of American troops from Vietnam and an end to a vicious, protracted war. Along with a half-dozen other "human torches," he is revered as a selfless *bodhisattva* by Vietnamese Buddhists.[1] His heart, seared by the blaze but still intact, is enshrined on the altar of Xa Loi Pagoda in Saigon.

One dawn on Chakpori Hill, just outside of Lhasa, the capital city of Tibet, a silent procession moves slowly to the top of a craggy barren mount. As the procession nears the "cemetery" atop the mound, members of a special class of morticians known as *rogyapa* (*ro rgya pa*, corpse cutters) clear a spot to place the body of an old man who passed away three days before. The body, wrapped in plain white cloth, has been carried on a stretcher accompanied by close friends, monks, and family members. At the head of the procession is a *thangka* (*thang ga*, religious scroll painting) depicting the *bodhisattva* Avalokitesvara fixed to a makeshift post. The *bodhisattva*, on behalf of the deceased, has been honored with a *khata* (*kha btags*), a traditional white scarf symbolizing purity and auspiciousness. Amidst the monks' prayers for a favorable rebirth, the body has been washed in fragrant herbs, then placed in the center of a prepared space and the cloth removed. After some time, the *rogyapas* begin their appointed task of chopping up the limbs of the body, pounding them, and mixing them with roasted barley flour to feed to the vultures that hover nearby. This kind of "sky burial" is the most common mode of disposing of the dead in Tibet, since the frozen ground and the lack of trees make both burial and cremation impractical. The time for disposing of the body is chosen through divination, conducted either by a *lama* (lit., teacher, a religious specialist), or an astrologer who determines when the consciousness has left the body. The rite serves as a stark reminder of the impermanence and interconnectedness of all life and is regarded as a final act of generosity by close relatives on behalf of the deceased.[2]

These two images of death and the associations they evoke reveal several paradoxes between doctrine and social practice in Buddhist cultures. All Buddhist traditions ultimately trace their roots to India and the teachings of Buddha Śākyamuni. Over hundreds of years, the fundamental teaching of the Buddha evolved into a rich variety of Buddhist traditions, each with its unique interpretations and practices. A variety of attitudes toward the body and consciousness, life and death, this world and the next, reflect not only the independent developments of the Buddha's teachings, but also the influences of indigenous thought and practice. Buddhist ideas about the nature of consciousness, the process of conscious dying, rebirth within different realms of existence, and liberation from cyclic existence were adapted in the process of interaction with local beliefs, rituals, and customs. The resulting eclectic blends of belief and practice are apparent in disparate Buddhist cultures today, especially in relation to death and dying. The variety of beliefs and practices associated with death in Buddhist cultures, especially in Tibet, provide new ways of looking at the universal experience of dying.

The Four Sights

When Siddhārtha Gautama first left his father's palace, he witnessed four sights that turned him to the spiritual quest: a sick person, an old person, a dead person, and a renunciant. Because his father, King

Śuddhodana, had conscientiously shielded him from unpleasant experiences, these four sights alerted the young prince to the realities of life and set him on the path to awakening. After his enlightenment, the Buddha taught his followers to reflect on these same realities in order to gain a better understanding about the human condition and the precariousness of life. According to the Buddha, reflection on death and impermanence is the key means to awakening from the slumber of ignorance, gaining insight into "things as they are," and achieving liberation from the wheel of birth and death.

The centrality of death and impermanence in Buddhist thought is evident in the texts of all Buddhist traditions. Sentient beings are portrayed as trapped in the cycle of birth and death like animals tangled in a net. Suffering (*dukkha*), impermanence (*anitya*), and no-self (*anātman*) are the three "marks" of cyclic existence. The term *duhkha* includes mental and physical sufferings, all dissatisfactions, and the all-encompassing unsatisfactory quality that characterizes the cycle of rebirth. As the Buddha described it:

> This, O Bhikkhus, is the Noble Truth of Suffering:
> Birth is suffering; decay is suffering;
> illness is suffering; death is suffering.[3]

Impermanence refers not only to death at the end of a lifetime, but also to the momentary process of production and disintegration that characterizes conditioned things. All that arises will inevitably perish, even the most minute particles that are the basis for presuming the existence of persons. Comprised of constantly shifting physical and mental elements, living beings are said to be dying from the moment they are born.

The inevitability of death is often illustrated by the story of Kisagotamī. A cousin of the Buddha, Kisagotamī went mad from the shock of losing her only child. Totally deranged, she carried the dead child's body from house to house in hopes of bringing him back to life. Eventually someone directed her to the Buddha and Kisagotamī pleaded with him to restore her child's life. The Buddha agreed to do it, on the one condition that she bring him a mustard seed from a house where no one had ever died. As she went from house to house, she soon realized that no one was untouched by death, and thus recovered her sanity. She later became an ordained nun and applied herself intensively to meditation practice. Eventually she achieved the state of an *arhat* and celebrated her attainment of *nirvāṇa*, "the undying," with this verse:

>I have practiced the Great Eightfold Way straight
> to the undying.
>I have come to the great peace.
>I have looked into the mirror of the Dharma.[4]

The reflections on death, impermanence, and suffering that were so
pivotal in the awakening of the Buddha and Kisagotamī are central to
the Buddhist worldview and to the Buddhist cultural legacy that has
been transmitted to lands far and wide. In each country, the Buddhist
reflections on death assume unique cultural expressions.

The Question of Rebirth

The Buddhists inherited or appropriated the doctrines of *karma* and
rebirth from earlier Indian thought. Buddha Śākyamuni affirmed these
doctrines, but reinterpreted them, replacing the belief in a soul with
teachings on impermanence, suffering, and soulessness. The perennial
question that arises is: If consciousness is insubstantial and impermanent, and there is no underlying soul or self, by what mechanism do
the impressions of virtuous and non-virtuous actions in one lifetime
bear fruit in another? In the early Buddhist texts, the continuity of
consciousness is likened to a flame that lights a candle, though nothing is transmitted from one to the other. No two moments of an
individual's stream of consciousness are the same, yet actions give rise
to consequences. This analogy is used to explain questions about the
relationship between actions and their effects, and about the relationship between one lifetime and the next. From a Buddhist viewpoint,
even without an underlying soul or self, an individual's actions in one
lifetime may have consequences in another. Although the stream of
consciousness in one life is neither the same nor different than the
stream that continues into the next, the imprints or potencies of actions imbue successive moments of consciousness with specific psychological tendencies. Just as personal identity continues from day to
day in one lifetime, even though no two moments are the same, Buddhists assume that a very subtle stream of causally connected moments of consciousness continues in future lifetimes.

Buddhists do not spend much time analyzing the claims and
assumptions about rebirth that prevailed when the Buddha taught. At
the time when Buddhism arose in India, the idea of life as a phase in
a continuous cycle of birth, death, and rebirth (*saṃsāra*) was already so
prevalent that little effort was spent formulating a convincing case for
rebirth. Further, Indian notions of infinite, cyclical time and infinite

world systems make speculation about the evolution of human consciousness and rebirth somewhat irrelevant, for the destruction of life in one world system does not mean the end of all life. Instead, Buddhist analysts direct their attention to the doctrine of no-self, the relationship between no-self and rebirth, and the ethical implications of *karma* and rebirth. Whether or not the theories of rebirth and no-self are convincing or mutually entailing, for Buddhists these assumptions have a significant impact on ethical decision making.

For Buddhism's critics, rebirth is impossible without an *ātman*, whereas for the Buddhists, the *anātman* theory is what makes rebirth possible. Only a mutable construct can undergo evolution, never a fixed one, since a static phenomenon is impervious to change. If the person who emerges in the next life is the same as in the past, no evolution is possible and hence no liberation. If the person who emerges in the next life is different from that in former lives, there is no necessary and contingent relationship between the former and the latter, so again no evolution is possible, and hence no liberation. The Buddhists use this logic to refute the notion of a core self as well as the notion of a radical discontinuity between moments. Instead they assert the theory of dependent arising and maintain that it is sufficient to explain causal continuities. All phenomena arise in dependence on their antecedent causes and on context, or conditions. The theory of dependent arising also serves to explain how sentient beings become trapped in the vicious cycle of *saṃsāra*. Ignorance gives rise to karmic formations, and sequentially to consciousness, name and form, the six sense powers, contact, feeling, clinging, grasping, existence, birth, and, finally, old age, and death. These topics, which elaborate on the basic doctrine of cause and effect, are recurrent themes in Buddhist texts and thinking.

Some Western scholars, such as Richard Hayes, contend that the theory of rebirth is unessential to Buddhist praxis: "It is not necessary to believe in rebirth to get benefit from Buddhist practices. One can still be liberated from greed, hatred, and delusion. And if one lives well on this side of the funeral pyre, then one will probably fare well in a future life, if there is one."[5] He maintains that "The doctrine of rebirth is an assumption that one holds independent of reason in order to sustain a set of ethical values."[6] This logic is useful for those who find Buddhist practice meaningful, but are not comfortable with the theory of rebirth. This should not obscure the fact that the stated goal of the Buddhist path is liberation from repeated rebirth. Disjoined from the theory of rebirth, the concept of liberation can only be taken allegorically. The theory of rebirth is integral to Buddhist soteriology;

repeated rebirth is the crucible for repeated, unimaginable suffering, so the central dilemma for living beings is how to end it once and for all.

Indian Roots of Buddhist Tradition

An examination of attitudes toward death in Buddhist cultures naturally leads back to an inquiry of early Indian Buddhist thought. Issues of death and personal identity have been central to the Buddha's teachings since the very beginning and have continued to be the focus of analysis and disputation for more than two and a half millennia. The concepts of death, impermanence, and personhood were an integral part of the Buddhist worldview that spread to Tibet and other lands in Asia, going in unprecedented directions in new cultural and philosophical climates. Indian Buddhist refutations of the notion of self or soul, for example, collided with indigenous Tibetan beliefs about multiple personal souls and Chinese beliefs about spirits and ghosts. The Buddha's emphasis on individual liberation and monastic practice came up against ancient customs that valued social interrelatedness, filial piety, and ancestral continuity. Local deities and beliefs had to somehow adjust and find their place in the Buddhist cosmological scheme.

Patterns of Buddhist accommodation to local beliefs and practices help explain the relatively rapid local acceptance gained by the new faith and cosmology. These patterns of accommodation extended to ways of thinking about death, raising numerous important philosophical and ethical questions that provide rich material for comparative analysis. A question arises, however: If there is no soul, and consciousness is momentary, what is it that travels from life to life? Consecutive moments of consciousness arise and cease incessantly like waves in the ocean, so how are the impressions of positive and negative actions (karma) transmitted from one lifetime to the next? Without the belief in a substantial self, what is the motivating force for ethical conduct and enlightenment? If living beings evolve over countless lifetimes, what does this mean for our understanding of death? These questions about the paradox of no-self and rebirth continue to engage scholars as Buddhism spreads to new lands and cultures right up to the present day.

Precisely what happens after the moment of death is a matter of ongoing dispute among Buddhists, yet all schools concur that ordinary beings somehow experience another existence. Whether the next birth (jāti) or re-existence (punabbhava) is pleasant or unpleasant depends upon one's previous actions (karma), wholesome or unwholesome. For example, Buddhaghoṣa's *Visuddhimagga* relates that when the life-continuum ends, an evil person is enveloped by the store of his or her evil deeds. First, the death consciousness arises and ceases, then the "rebirth-linking" consciousness arises, and due to the negative *karma* previously created, the unfortunate signs of an unhappy destiny (the flames of hell, forests of knives, etc.) appear.[7] Conversely, when the life-continuum ends, a virtuous person is enveloped by his or her good deeds. After the death consciousness arises and ceases, the rebirth-linking consciousness arises, and due to the positive *karma* previously created, the pleasant signs of a happy destiny (pleasure groves, heavenly palaces, wish-fulfilling trees, etc.) appear.[8]

Buddhaghoṣa, the foremost commentator in the Pāli tradition, describes how like gives rise to like: the material (*rūpa*, form) gives rise to the material, while the immaterial (*vijñāna*, consciousness) gives rise to the immaterial. In accordance with dependent arising (*pratītyasamutpāda*), the life-continuum begins from the "rebirth-linking" consciousness and continues until the death consciousness at the end of the life span.[9] At the time of death, one "puts down" or leaves behind the corporeal aggregates of the previous life and assumes or "takes up" the corporeal aggregates that begin the next life continuum. All the "formations" between birth and death—the varied experiences of life—are characterized by impermanence (*anitya*), unsatisfactoriness (*dukkha*), and no-soul (*anātman*). The "formations" are described as being no-self or soulless, because they are devoid of self or "ownerless."[10] The life span is divided into ten stages: "the tender decade, the sport decade, the beauty decade," and so on, with the formations disintegrating all the while and life careening uncontrollably toward its inevitable conclusion. The various stages of life are therefore in a ceaseless process of formation and disintegration from moment to moment. The Indian Buddhist perspective on life and death is congruous with its perspective on the bipolar modality of phenomena: a thing can be either permanent or impermanent; there is no third alternative. Therefore, if a self were to exist, it would have to be either a permanent phenomena or an impermanent phenomenon. Buddhaghoṣa vigorously denies that any component of the being is transmitted from one life to the next, and his view is commonly held by Theravāda Buddhist practitioners today. The Pāli texts go to great lengths to establish that the "self," like all conditioned things, is impermanent and lacking in any permanent core.

In the *Abhidharmakośa*, Vasubandhu describes an intermediate being (*antarābhāva*) in an transitional state of indeterminate length. The intermediate being is said to be visible only to certain beings, possessed of complete sense faculties, and unimpeded by material obstacles. A being in the intermediate state lacks material substance, but nevertheless has a form which, although not visible to ordinary human beings, may be visible to other *bardo* beings, highly realized beings, and beings with the special capacity to perceive them. Because the intermediate being is impervious to material obstructions, it is able to travel through walls, mountains, and similar barriers. Such a being possesses complete sense faculties and is able to see, hear, smell, taste, feel sensations, and cognize. The being lacks materiality,[11] but still has the aggregates that are the basis for imputing the existence of a self. The ultimate destiny of the being is determined by its actions (karma) in previous lifetimes, that is, the nature of that being's future migration is dependent upon causes and conditions. Only one who has practiced intensively in preparation for the transition that occurs at death and gained sufficient mental control is capable of exerting an influence on its future state of existence or avoiding rebirth altogether by achieving liberation.

Buddhist Seeds on New Ground

Understandings of personal identity in the face of death shifted with the introduction of Buddhism into new lands and cultures in significant ways. The clash of values between family obligations and celibate monastic life in China, for example, is well-documented. Questions also arose around the concept of individual moral responsibility in a society that valued interpersonal relatedness and ancestral continuity. The Buddhist ideas that reached these new lands from India were not adopted unquestioningly, but underwent centuries of interpretation and adaptation in a variety of cultural environments. Not only were a variety of Buddhist texts, lineages, and philosophical streams received from India, but they sometimes arrived several centuries apart, taking new forms as they were planted on different cultural soil, and were nourished by different social, political, and intellectual ideas. The Buddhist traditions that developed in these countries became embedded in the larger Buddhist philosophical narrative, but were simultaneously situated within disparate cultural milieus and influenced by indigenous values, history, and custom. The results were a multiplicity of distinctive Buddhist philosophical and cultural traditions.

There were, of course, resemblances among the cultures that adopted Buddhist beliefs. For instance, as we examine early historical documents, we discover striking similarities between the shamanic worldviews and ritual practices found in China and Tibet prior to the introduction of Buddhism. In these early cultures, the boundaries between the seen and the unseen, this world and other worlds of experience were more fluid and permeable than in the modern scientific view. Human beings acknowledged and interacted with a pantheon of visible and invisible denizens of the cosmos: deities, demons, adversaries, and allies. Among the agriculturalists and pastoralists that inhabited these territories, ritual specialists and diviners communicated with unseen forces and were trusted to manipulate cosmic forces for fertility, protection, and healing.

In addition to shamanic beliefs and rituals, early Buddhist cultures also accommodated to indigenous explanations of life, death, and the human situation. The distinctive Buddhist cultural variants that resulted were reflections of differences in geography, language, and cultural history. Indigenous cultures served as the bedrock for a wealth of Buddhist cultural expressions and their influences are evident to the present day.

Buddhist texts did not reach China and Tibet in any systematic way, but were transmitted in different languages to different places, where they were translated and interpreted in a variety of ways. Sometimes more advanced texts and commentaries arrived from India and Central Asia earlier than the texts on which they were based, causing confusion and creative interpretation. The materials that were received and composed were imposing not only in terms of sheer numbers, but also in terms of philosophical complexity. Translating the Dharma into local languages involved creating new idioms to convey new ideas, an elaborate process that required centuries in China, Tibet, and Southeast Asia. This historical process gradually gave rise to unique philosophical perspectives on living and dying.

For example in China, Buddhist ideas were adopted into a complex cosmological schema of values and rituals. Ancient Chinese views on death and personal identity were never catalogued systematically and must be gleaned from an extensive corpus of literature including the Yijing and works attributed to Laozi, Confucius, Zhuangzi, and other early Chinese thinkers. This tapestry of ideas formed the backdrop against which Buddhist ideas from India were understood as they were introduced from the fourth century on. Upon the preexisting Chinese system of beliefs and ritual practices were grafted Buddhist ideas of rebirth, evolution within various realms of existence, ideas of impermanence and suffering, and a soteriology of personal liberation. And from this fusion of philosophical, moral, and religious convictions, uniquely Chinese rituals and funerary practices developed. For example, such ceremonies as the ghost festival, where the souls of the dead, along with personal items needed in the other world, are "crossed over" to a more auspicious rebirth, combine both imported Buddhist and indigenous beliefs.

In Tibet, a variety of Buddhist philosophical tenets, ethical codes, and meditation practices were transmitted from India, especially around the seventh century, and were grafted onto pre-Buddhist beliefs and practices. Shamanic beliefs and ritual practices within Bön cosmology, for example, dealt with personal protective deities and the transmigration of souls, or spirits, after death. As these beliefs and practices coexisted with Buddhist beliefs about death, an elaborate technology for negotiating the stages of the dying process gradually emerged. As Buddhaghoṣa explained in the *Visuddhimagga*, nothing solid continues after death, yet one moment of consciousness gives rise to the next. After the physical elements disintegrate, unless one has achieved a very high level of spiritual attainment and can consciously determine one's next state of existence, rebirth takes place as a result of karma and delusions. In line with the earliest Buddhist teachings, Tibetan scholars rejected the idea of a self that continues after death, yet they accepted the idea of a very subtle consciousness that continues into an intermediate state (*bardo*) between death and the next life. This led to the practice of recognizing the rebirth of highly regarded religious figures (*tulkus*) and eventually to rule by reincarnation, a system of religious institutional authority that provided political leadership in Tibet for centuries.

Hundreds of years have now passed since the introduction of Buddhism to distant lands and Indian Buddhist ideas have become so thoroughly integrated into the cultural fabrics of these countries that it is often difficult to determine what is distinctively Buddhist and what is not. From the Buddhist commentaries written by Chinese and Tibetan scholars, it is possible to discern similarities and differences of interpretation and emphasis. For example, the two traditions similarly emphasize the *bodhisattva* ideal, but practice different lineages of *bodhisattva* precepts. Core Buddhist principles may also be expressed differently in daily life. For example, to avoid taking life is a core Buddhist tenet, but Buddhists may interpret it differently. In Tibet, Buddhists are careful to avoid killing even the smallest insect, but they may have a lenient attitude toward eating meat. In China, many Buddhists are strictly vegetarian, but they may have a lenient attitude toward dispatching mosquitoes.

Self-immolation and sky burial illustrate an extreme contrast in interpretations. In 1982, when I visited Putoushan, the sacred site of the Avalokiteśvara, the Bodhisattva of Compassion, a sign was posted that read, "Please do not immolate yourself here." Another sign admonished, "Sacrifice of fingers and other body parts prohibited." Although self-immolation and self-mutilation are prohibited by law in the People's Republic of China, there is a long history of acts of physical sacrifice in China and the Chinese cultural diaspora, including Japan, Korea, and Vietnam. The practice of self-immolation is based on examples of self-sacrifice, such as those found in the *Saddharmapuṇḍarīka Sūtra*, a popular Mahāyāna text. Because the practice involves violence and a breach of the precept against taking life, it is not widely practiced. But what explains the prestige of the practice of physical sacrifice today when a traditional respect for physical integrity causes many Chinese to oppose organ transplantation?

Although the *Saddharmapuṇḍarīka Sūtra* is known in Tibet, self-immolation was not practiced there. The ideal of sacrificing the body for the welfare of sentient beings contained in this and many other *sūtras* is well known, but there is no record that the Tibetans took it literally. Still, in their zeal to achieve enlightenment as quickly as possible, some *yogis* are sealed into small retreat huts, where they live and die in total isolation, often leaving just their hair and fingernails behind. Although there is no custom of self-immolation in Tibet, there is a seemingly gruesome practice called *chö* (*chod*) in which the practitioner visualizes donating his or her own body parts to benefit sentient beings. These practices at once reflect Indian Buddhist beliefs and also suggest influences from indigenous belief and practices. Buddhist views on no-self, emptiness, and rebirth had to be understood in relation to earlier beliefs about spirits, souls, and the afterlife. Among ordinary Tibetans, there is a lingering belief in a personal soul, one that can be lost and recovered, which exists simultaneously with the *anātman* theory. The intersections that occurred in the philosophical and religious developments of these unique cultures undoubtedly gave rise to numerous conflicts of values and authority that can barely be distinguished through the shoals of time. The new Buddhist cosmology and human beings' place within it alternately converged and collided with earlier understandings until eventually comfortable permutations evolved. In these new environments, fresh insights and rituals emerged.

Buddhists in East Asia generally adopt the basic ethical framework established during the Buddha's time, including the core precept to refrain from taking life. In conjunction, they traditionally observe Confucian cultural taboos against destroying, dismembering, or disfiguring the body. This orientation is reflected in low rates of organ donation in East Asian societies (and Hawai'i) even today. The proscription against taking life may deter some individuals from the practice of suicide or self-destruction, yet Buddhists in these societies are familiar with the stories of self-sacrifice found in such texts as the *Saddharmapuṇḍarīka Sūtra* or the *Jātaka* stories of Buddha Śākyamuni's past lives.

In one *Jātaka* tale, for example, the Buddha offers his flesh to save a starving tigress and her cubs. A ritual of self-sacrifice is enacted by Buddhists in these countries during *bodhisattva* ordinations even today. Receiving three or more burns on the head is an integral part of the full ordination ceremony for Chinese nuns and monks, outlawed in mainland China only since 1982; the ritual symbolizes sacrificing one's body and even one's life for the sake of all sentient beings. Although we have no record of self-immolation among Buddhists in India, examples of practitioners burning their fingers, arms, or even their entire body as offerings to the Buddha, are well documented in China. In Vietnam, which was under Chinese rule for a thousand years and strongly influenced by Chinese Buddhism, the practice of self-immolation apparently began in 455 CE with the monk Tanhong and continued up to the immolations of Thich Quang Duc and others protesting the oppression of Buddhists in the 1960s. These practices have no counterpart in Tibetan Buddhist culture.

Likewise, the Tibetan practice of sky burial has no counterpart among Chinese Buddhists, who generally find the practice abhorrent. In recent years, the Chinese authorities in Tibet began turning sky burial into a tourist attraction, making a spectacle of what the Chinese regard as a barbaric practice. The attempt to sensationalize the Tibetan religious rite was finally discontinued after an international outcry and charges of cultural exploitation. From a Tibetan point of view, the rite has profound religious significance. Sky burial takes place after a religious specialist (*lama*) with a special talent for divination determines that the consciousness of the deceased has left the corpse and after the prescribed prayers, readings, and rituals have been performed. For Tibetans, to dismember the corpse and distribute it to birds and wild animals is not savage, but a deeply meaningful, spiritual act. The ritual not only helps bring closure to human relationships, but also benefits the deceased through the giving of food to numerous living beings. Because of the difficulty of burial in the frozen Tibetan soil and the dearth of firewood for cremation, distributing parts of the corpse in a final act of generosity is not considered macabre but rather a symbol of the dissolution that awaits all living things at death. Since generosity is the first of the six perfections (*pāramitā*), practices of central value for the *bodhisattva* on the Mahāyāna path, sky burial is regarded as a virtuous solution to a practical dilemma.

The Buddhist texts and commentaries explain the Buddha's teaching on the three characteristics of existence: unsatisfactoriness (*duhkha*), impermanence (*anitya*), and no-self (*anātman*), the lack of an enduring, independently existing self or soul. These texts may have been little known outside the monasteries and likely exerted little influence on common folk, but Buddhist ideas and values have exerted a great influence on these cultures for hundreds of years. While attempting to preserve the original Buddhist teachings from India, each culture developed its own distinctive interpretations and cultural practices that express them. The practices of self-immolation and sky burial reveal different cultural attitudes toward death, the integrity of the body, and the relationships between individuals and communities. It is difficult to overestimate how thoroughly the teachings of the Buddha have permeated the thinking and lives of the people in Buddhist cultures. In Japan, the falling of cherry blossoms in spring is enough to convey volumes on the philosophy of impermanence. Because Buddhist cultures share so much common ground, their unique attitudes and customs are a convenient starting point for understanding the diverse beliefs and cultural practices that arose in response to death.

Philosophical Foundations

Mahāyāna texts further elaborated the theory of no-self in terms of the two levels of truth, explaining the self as conventionally existent, but empty of any independent reality. This interpretation is consistent with the earliest Buddhist teachings about the absence of any soul or abiding identity, yet allows for the ripening of an individual's karma over the course of many rebirths. Both the Madhyamaka and Yogācāra branches of Mahāyāna incorporate these fundamental understandings of Buddhist tenets.

The majority of Tibetan Buddhist scholars adopt Chandrakrti's radical deconstructionist approach to Madhyamaka which denies any inherent identity to self and phenomena. When H. H. Dalai Lama was asked at the Waikiki Shell in 1994, "What happens to us after we die?" he quipped, "Generally speaking, we are no more." This response is typical of the Madhyamaka view most famously presented in the *Prajñāhṛdaya Sūtra* (*Heart of Wisdom Sūtra*): "There is no form, no sound, no smell, no taste, no tactile object, no phenomenon. . . . There is no ignorance and no exhaustion of ignorance, and so forth up to no aging and death and no exhaustion of aging and death." The illusory self, which exists conventionally and dependently, on the basis of its component parts, simply ceases to exist when those parts are rent asunder.

In the Yogācāra school that became prominent in China, external phenomena are viewed as mere manifestations of mind. This view also neutralizes the tendency to concretize the self, though in a different way. The difficult question about how the imprints of actions (*karma*) continue to exert an influence over the course of several lifetimes is also addressed in a new way. An additional "storehouse" consciousness, called the *ālayavijñāna*, is identified to act as a repository of karmic imprints, to explain how the results of our actions are experienced beyond death.

The different philosophical approaches to the nature of reality presented in the Madhyamaka and Yogācāra schools suggest different interpretations of personal identity and its dissolution at the time of death. Each school has its own ways to explain how the impact of actions carries over through the seemingly endless round of rebirths. The challenge is to reconcile the theory of karma—the basis of Buddhist ethics—with the theory of rebirth without falling into the fallacy of self. To investigate whether, and in what ways, different interpretations of the philosophical tenets of these schools account for different understandings of consciousness, death, personal identity, and moral agency, especially as they relate to bioethical concerns, it is necessary to thoroughly understand Buddhism's roots in India.

Buddhas, Bodhisattvas, and Ordinary Beings

A further topic to consider is what death means to a *bodhisattva* or a Buddha. Do *bodhisattvas* and Buddhas die like ordinary mortals or are they beyond death? What does death mean for an embodied Buddha such as Śākyamuni who has transcended discursive thought? What does it mean for a *bodhisattva* who willingly defers liberation for the good of the world? Does the *bodhisattva* ideal contribute to the illusion of self or undermine it? To strive for Buddhahood requires not only much dedication and conviction, but also tremendous self-confidence, even pride: "I vow to liberate all beings without exception, to take upon myself the responsibility for establishing each and every one in the state of perfect Buddhahood." Is the wish to liberate all living beings a form of self-effacement or is it, as Trungpa Rinpoche once remarked, "the biggest ego trip that ever happened?"

In the early Buddhist texts, a Buddha like Śākyamuni is portrayed as an ordinary human being who, through diligent practice, achieves the state of *nirvāṇa* and passes away ("enters *parinirvāṇa*"), more or less like any other person, although perhaps with more equanimity and wisdom. Prior to enlightenment, a *bodhisattva* is a selfless practitioner who aims at liberating all sentient beings, but is otherwise vulnerable to death and rebirth, just like everyone else. As the Mahāyāna teachings evolved, these concepts begin to change as the Buddhas and *bodhisattvas* progressively take on more mythic proportions.

Even in pre-Mahāyāna texts, a practitioner who successfully attains the state of a fully enlightened Buddha is no longer subject to birth and death and is therefore liberated from cyclic existence (*saṃsāra*). The Mahāyāna texts explicitly state that one who has achieved the status of a *bodhisattva* has also achieved the power to determine one's future rebirth. Unlike ordinary beings who are "thrown" to the next rebirth propelled by *karma* and afflictive emotions, a *bodhisattva* achieves the power to emanate multiple bodies in multiple world systems in order to benefit sentient beings. The motivating force behind the *bodhisattva*'s endeavors is not pride or egotism, but boundless compassion.

In Tibet, the belief in the *bodhisattvas*' power to reincarnate intentionally became institutionalized in the *tulku* system, in which reincarnate *lamas* are recognized in childhood, revered as being the reembodiments of specific highly realized practitioners, and singled out for special treatment and education. The word "*tulku*" is the Tibetan translation of the Sanskrit word "*nirmāṇakāya*," signifying the emanation body in the *trikāya* theory of the Buddha. The oldest *tulku* lineage, that of the Karmapas, began with Tüsum Khyenpa (1110–1193) and continues until the present, with the seventeenth Karmapa, Ugyen Trinley Dorje, who recently escaped Chinese domination and defected to India.

Unlike the *bodhisattvas* who intentionally take rebirth in *saṃsāra* to benefit sentient beings, Buddhas are viewed as perfectly enlightened beings whose enlightened activities benefit sentient beings through emanations that do not require taking an ordinary birth. For this reason, the texts refer to the ultimate attainment of Buddhahood as having achieved the deathless *dharmakāya*, the formless, enlightened wisdom aspect of a Buddha. These various identities and permutations within the various Buddhist traditions are, like all phenomena, ultimately devoid of abiding identity. Whereas the enlightened awareness of a Buddha is permanent, on the conventional level, Buddhas, *bodhisattvas*, *arhats*, and ordinary beings alike are identity-less, operating on a ceaselessly changing, conventional level of reality. Even the *bodhisattva*, who is recognized as the reembodiment of a spiritual adept, manifesting the predispositions of an earlier incarnation, represents simply another phase in a continuous series of conventional identities.

Chapter 3

Understanding the Nature of Consciousness

When Buddhists approach the topics of death and ethical decision making, their primary focus is not the body or soul, but consciousness. Consciousness is central to human experience, because it is the means by which we know the world around us. There are many different Buddhist philosophical perspectives, but generally speaking, existing things belong to three mutually exclusive categories: matter, consciousness, and "non-associated factors" (things that are neither matter nor consciousness, like undifferentiated space). Phenomena—the things around us—exist insofar as they are objects of knowledge, established by valid cognition.

The Buddha taught a path to liberation for all sentient beings, meaning beings with consciousness: human beings, animals, and many other life forms. All sentient beings are involved in the wheel of birth and death known as cyclic existence (saṃsāra). Since the beginning of time (or beginningless time, as the Buddhists put it), countless beings have been migrating from one state of existence to another in accordance with the law of cause and effect or, as some texts put it, "at the mercy of karma and delusion." Sentient beings continue to take birth again and again, sometimes in blissful states of existence and sometimes in truly miserable states of existence, depending on their previous actions. The goal for Buddhists is to free themselves from this repetitive, seemingly endless cycle of rebirths, that is, to achieve liberation. The key to gaining liberation from the cycle of rebirth is to purify the mind of all afflictions, such as greed, attachment, anger, hatred, and ignorance, and thereby avoid creating unwholesome deeds.

To understand how living beings become caught up in cyclic existence and how they can become free from it, an understanding of the nature and functioning of consciousness is therefore essential.

By consciousness, Buddhists simply mean knowing or awareness. Consciousness is not a solid or enduring entity, but simply an impermanent stream or continuity of conscious moments. Each moment of consciousness gives rise to a subsequent moment of consciousness, in accordance with the law of cause and effect. These conscious events—mental or sensory—continue from moment to moment like a string of pearls, each moment giving rise to the next. Even during sleep, the continuum of consciousness is present in a subtle form.

At each moment of each lifetime, conscious awareness is the process through which sentient beings experience happiness, unhappiness, and many other emotions and perceptions. Consciousness is just one of the elements that comprise the human being, but it is the most important one, because it is the central processing center for all experiences. At the moment of death, consciousness is also present and is critical in the process of taking another rebirth. The last moment of awareness in one lifetime acts as the cause of the next moment of awareness, which is the first moment of the next state of existence. Understanding the nature of consciousness is thus crucial for understanding the process of dying and rebirth.

In the Buddhist schema, there are six different types of consciousness. The five sense consciousnesses arise in dependence on the sense faculties or powers (*indriya*) and mental consciousness arises in dependence on the mental faculty or power. When one of the five sense faculties (eye, ear, nose, tongue, or body) comes into contact with its respective sense object, a moment of sense consciousness (visual, auditory, olfactory, gustatory, tactile, or mental) comes into being. When the mental faculty comes into contact with a thought or mental image, a moment of mental consciousness comes into being. The continually changing series of conscious mental events constitutes the mental continuum. Sense experience—seeing, hearing, smelling, tasting, and touching—is subsequently processed through the mental faculty, which labels, distinguishes, and acts on it. The duration of each moment of consciousness is brief, perhaps one-seventy-fifth of a second, a theory supported by recent findings in experimental psychology. In addition to the six types of primary consciousness, the texts describe more than fifty mental factors.

The terms "consciousness" (*jñāna*), awareness (*buddhi*), and knowing (*saṃvedana*) are used synonymously. These terms are generally preferred to the term "mind," which may connote something more solid or enduring. The term consciousness is also used to denote the mental continuum—a sequence of impermanent, dependently arising moments of awareness (*citta*). The idea of a self-reflective consciousness—that is, a consciousness that is aware of consciousness—is rejected by most Buddhist schools. One is simply aware, moment to moment. The idea of an underlying foundation or substratum of consciousness is also rejected, except in the later Yogācāra system.

Consciousness is not necessarily conceptual. A moment of visual awareness, for example, is also a moment of consciousness. The mind is capable of being aware of many different sights, sounds, smells, tastes, and tactile sensations, and many different mental perceptions, though only one at a time. Human beings receive an enormous amount of data through the senses, moment to moment, and process it mentally, often without conscious intent. Once the data is received, it is then processed conceptually, and that is where problems begin.

A moment of consciousness may be either a moment of direct perception (*pratyakṣha*) or of conceptual cognition. Conceptual cognition is of two types: inferential cognition (*anumānapramāṇa*) and subsequent cognition (*parichchhinna-jñana*). Awareness of direct (nonconceptual) perception, whether direct sense perception or direct mental perception requires conscientious training. The first moment of perception is said to be nonconceptual; the second and subsequent moments of perception are conceptual and, therefore, necessarily instances of mental consciousness. Neither mental nor sense perception is possible without the mental faculty. Although the sense faculties and the mental faculty are not physical in nature, they are associated with physical sense organs. The relationship between sense faculties, sense objects, sense perceptions, and mental perceptions is the subject of an ongoing dialogue between Buddhists and neurophysicists about the relationship between mind and brain.[1]

The way that our mental consciousness processes the sensory impressions of phenomena around us, and the mental impressions of phenomena within our own minds, has a great deal to do with the way we interpret and respond to those phenomena. If our consciousness is cluttered with self-interest, preconceptions, and projections, our knowing and thinking will be distorted. This can distort the way we react to events, leading to many mistakes, misunderstandings, and misfortunes. For Buddhists, these difficulties do not affect just one lifetime, but carry forward into future lifetimes as well. After the dissolution of the physical constituents of an individual at death, the momentary stream of consciousness continues to another rebirth and is imbued with the tendencies or propensities created by actions in the past. The quality of one's consciousness and one's actions are therefore of critical concern, because they sow the seeds that propel us to the next state of existence.

In Buddhist thought, the elements that constitute a sentient being are all mutable and fleeting. A person exists conventionally, based on the physical and psychological component that constitute the person, but there is no element of the person that exists permanently or ultimately. There can be little disagreement that the physical components of the person disintegrate or are reduced to ashes after death. However, what becomes of the psychological components of a person at death, if anything, is a matter of speculation. Buddhists generally agree that the momentary stream of consciousness continues into another state of existence, in dependence on actions (karma) and the law of cause and effect. However, among the Buddhists of different traditions, opinions differ about how this process occurs and exactly what becomes of a being's stream of consciousness after death.

Consciousness and Individual Identity

The mutable nature of consciousness and the other components of personal identity challenges the ordinary human tendency to reify phenomena. Whether we use the term self, or ego, or personal identity, for Buddhists it is precisely the notion of an enduring entity that is the root cause of suffering. The mutable nature of phenomena comes into conflict with the hope that our self will endure. When we look for the self, in contemplation, it is impossible to identify any enduring entity that meets that description. Yet the belief in an enduring, independently existing self is very strong, and it leads to many anxieties, disappointments, and problems.

The very fact that human beings are constantly reconstructing and redefining themselves demonstrates how amorphous and unsatisfactory the concept of self-identify is, but attachment to the self is very powerful and can even be overwhelming. Clinging to the self results in feelings of anger and unhappiness when things do not go our way or threaten our cherished image of our self. The more strongly we cling to our self-image, the more intensely we suffer when the physical body ages, falls ill, and eventually comes to an end. Death is the greatest suffering of all, because it is the ultimate threat to our self-identity and self-interest. As long as we cling to ourselves or our loved ones, death brings great suffering. But when we analyze the notion of self and try to identify an independently existing self, we cannot find one. The notion that dying is a tragedy is therefore based on a false premise. Death may be tragic, but not in the way we ordinarily imagine.

When human beings face death, they usually encounter a number of unpleasant experiences. Terminal illness not only can bring raw physical suffering, but also the suffering of loneliness, poverty, and anxiety. In addition, the end of life brings the sufferings of unfulfilled expectations and the unhappiness of having to leave our loved ones and possessions behind. The unfamiliar setting of a hospital can cause disorientation, anger, and frustration. Although reason tells us that we will be stripped of all possessions, we still worry about expenses. At the end of life, we face the loss of our very self-identity, which gives rise to uncertainty and fear. We have no choice but to reconcile ourselves to the inevitability of death, however, we must also resign ourselves to not knowing the time of death, the nature of death, or what lies beyond death.

It is commonly assumed that theories about an eternal soul that survives death are designed to allay the fear of death in human beings, but fear and doubt about the afterlife can also become a source of anxiety. The belief in an enduring soul can lead to clinging and grasping at the self, and enhance the illusion of a permanent identity, which can lead to further fear and suffering when the body and mental faculties begin to deteriorate. The irritation we feel as our memory deteriorates and the anger that often attends dementia are symptomatic of our attachment to our failing mental and physical competence.

Consciousness and Repeated Becoming

This present life is very short and fragile, but future lives are innumerable. Because all living beings have created innumerable actions, both wholesome and unwholesome, the circumstances of our future states of rebirth is uncertain. The mechanics of rebirth and the nature of the linkage between the different states of existence are very subtle and open to interpretation, but the process is definitely related to consciousness. Buddhists are principally concerned with consciousness, because the environments within which sentient beings take rebirth are dependent upon their actions (*karma*) and their actions are dependent upon consciousness. Liberation from the wheel of *karma* and rebirth therefore depends on the purification of mental consciousness.

When the conceptual faculty is clouded by desires, aversions, ignorance, and other mental afflictions, these mental afflictions obscure our ability to know things accurately. If the mental consciousness can be purified of the mental afflictions that distort the way we know things, then we can avoid many problems and painful experiences. Understanding the nature of the mind and how it functions is essential for recognizing how we create both happiness and problems for ourselves and other living beings. Understanding the nature of the mind and purifying it is the central focus of the Buddhist teachings.

Indian Buddhist texts make a distinction between calm abiding meditation (śamatha) and insight meditation (vipaśyanā). Calm abiding meditation trains the mind to remain tranquil, focused, and collected, using the faculty of concentration to settle the mind calmly on one object. Insight meditation trains the mind using the faculty of analysis to reflect and investigate matters in order to develop understanding. The goal of these contemplations is to develop insight into the true nature of things, namely, the unsatisfactory (duhkha), impermanent (anitya), and no-self (anātman) nature of all phenomena. These general rubrics encompass a range of practices that can be very useful in life and especially at the end of life. Mindfulness (sati) is a practice of being alert to whatever arises in one's field of experience, moment to moment. This practice of being fully attentive, each and every moment, helps one maintain awareness and equanimity, no matter what happens. There are also meditations that act as antidotes to particular disturbing emotions; for example, meditation on patience to transform anger, generosity to transform stinginess, and loving kindness to transform hatred. Contemplation on the Buddha's teachings is also considered practice. Reflecting on the teachings helps people deal with daily frustrations and also helps them prepare for the experiences of sickness, aging, and dying. For example, contemplation on suffering leads to the realization that suffering is universal to all sentient beings—an insight that counteracts any sense of victimization. The wisdom that recognizes old age and death as natural phases of life helps one cope with these unpleasant realities. Likewise, the wisdom that understands the nature of consciousness as momentary helps prepare one for the transition from one lifetime to the next. In all these ways, meditation and contemplation can be both useful and liberating.

In most Buddhist schools, matter and consciousness are two distinct categories and causal connectedness operates separately within these two broad categories. Functional phenomena are produced by causes similar in nature to themselves (samanantarapratyaya): material causes give rise to material results and moments of consciousness give rise to subsequent moments of consciousness. Physical matter and consciousness are interconnected and often contingent, but are phenomenologically distinct categories. All functional phenomena, whether matter or consciousness, are momentary, arising in dependence on causes and conditions. Phenomena exist conventionally and can be named, but do not exist ultimately. In the Buddhist view, the five sense consciousnesses arise in dependence upon contact between the five sense faculties (eye, ear, nose, tongue, and body) and their respective objects. The sixth type of consciousness, mental consciousness, arises in dependence upon the mental faculty, which is not physical. To assert that consciousness discontinues at death is to assume that consciousness cannot exist independently of a physical foundation, and there is no evidence to support this view. Although it has been shown that certain mental functions are dependent on specific areas of the brain, there is no evidence that consciousness is identical to the brain. If it is possible to show that any aspect of consciousness is not dependent upon the brain, then it is possible that this aspect of consciousness can continue after the physical body disintegrates at death.[2]

Although the mental consciousness is not directly dependent upon the body, it is closely related, because the data received by the senses is labeled and evaluated by the mental consciousness. Because Buddhists generally regard matter and consciousness as different categories of phenomena, they are not faced with the mind-body problem that arises from separating mental and physical experience, or from privileging the mental. When one examines the aggregate of consciousness for evidence of a self, one finds only a momentary stream of causally connected conscious events. On the basis of this series of causally connected conscious events, human beings assume the existence of a solid identity, when in fact there is nothing to back up this assumption.

Buddhist discussions about death are specifically concerned with the death of sentient beings, not with the death of plants or other non-sentient things. The reason is that, in the majority view, only beings with consciousness are capable of conscious evolution and enlightenment. The definition of enlightenment is the awakening of consciousness, so to achieve liberation, enlightenment, or awakening, one must possess sentience, or consciousness. The central goal of the Buddhist path is to eliminate suffering and plants, as far as we know, do not feel pain. Plants have life and may respond to stimuli, but they are not included in the category of sentient life because they lack conscious awareness and are therefore incapable of achieving the goals of the Buddhist path. Although later Mahāyāna Buddhists in East Asia express a wish to liberate "every blade of grass," this sentiment is not mentioned in Indian Buddhist texts. Consciousness simply means knowing and awareness. Although consciousness may become temporarily obscured or defiled by the afflictive emotions, it is not inherently defiled and therefore has the potential for awakening. All sentient beings have the capacity to purify their minds by removing these temporary defilements and to thereby achieve liberation.

Certainly, there is a close relationship between mind and body, but until recently it was unclear what that relationship was. Now significant progress is being made to understand the activity of the brain and its relationship to stress, depression, anxiety, and other psychological disorders. Neurophysicists, neurobiologists, and neuropsychologists are also beginning to document the medical benefits of meditation in clinical studies. In a new study, Richard Davidson at the University of Wisconsin and Jon Kabat-Zinn at the University of Massachusetts Medical School present findings about what happens in the brain during meditation.[3] Their work indicates a correlation between stress levels and the activity of the right and left sections of the frontal cortex of the brain. People with greater activity in the left frontal cortex of the brain tend to be calm and easygoing, whereas people with overactivity in the right frontal cortex tend to be anxious or depressed. These differences seem to be related not only to emotional well-being, but also to the functioning of the immune system and therefore physical health. In studies on the brain-wave function of control groups of meditators and non-meditators, collected from EEGs, researchers found shifts between the left and right frontal lobes and also differences in immune response. Studies by Solomon Snyder and neuroscientists at Johns Hopkins School of Medicine suggest that meditation practice increases the level of the calming neurotransmitter serotonin.

Although there is still much work to be done before the precise relationship between the brain, consciousness, and the nervous system can be known, neuroscientists are making significant contributions by studying the effects of meditation. Perhaps one day they will be able to determine precisely the nature of consciousness and to explain how consciousness enters the body. Buddhists generally accept the theory that consciousness continues from one lifetime to the next, based not on clinical studies, but on meditation experience. They find no convincing reason to assume that consciousness ends at death except that death is beyond ordinary human experience. If the continuity of consciousness from one lifetime to the next could be verified through direct experience in meditation, it would still be difficult to verify that type of yogic experience scientifically.

Human beings normally identify with their bodies, experiences, and activities uncritically, without questioning the nature of that identification. Many believe that the mind dies when the body does, whereas others believe that there is either some physical continuity in the afterlife or at least some continuity of identity, such as spirit or soul. In the traditional Buddhist schema, by contrast, the physical body and consciousness, though closely interrelated, are two separate categories

of phenomena. There is a continuity, but it is only the causally produced continuity of a very subtle level of consciousness, not a soul or
any substantial entity. In the Buddhist view, both the material elements of the body and nonmaterial elements of consciousness are
produced by causes similar to themselves. No substratum of identity
is required for creatures to live and die. Like all conditioned things,
sentient beings are momentary. They come into being, function for some
time, and disintegrate, all as a result of causes and conditions. Precisely
because there is no fixed substrate, the physical and conscious components of sentient beings arise, perish, and become transformed.

Francis Crick advances "The Astonishing Hypothesis" that human beings—their joys, sorrows, memories, ambitions, sense of personal identity, and free will—are nothing more than "the behavior of
a vast assembly of nerve cells and their associated molecules."[4] This
model explains consciousness solely in terms of physical causes and
effects, and asserts that consciousness cannot exist independently of a
living physical organism. In the Buddhist model, by contrast, physical
phenomena are distinct from mental phenomena, even though they
are interrelated and equally subject to the law of cause and effect.
Crick's model assumes that consciousness must necessarily be associated with a physical body, whereas the Buddhist model assumes that
consciousness can exist apart from a physical body. Although body
and mind are ordinarily thought of as interdependent, this is not
necessarily the case. A corpse is an example of a body that exists
without consciousness. In the Buddhist schema, beings in the formless
realm (*ārūpyadhātu*) are examples of beings with only mental consciousness, existing independently of a physical body.[5]

Consciousness and Continuity

In the *Pramanavarttika*, Dharmakīrti explains why matter is an insufficient cause for consciousness. Consciousness, being a compounded
phenomenon, must have a cause similar in nature to itself, that is,
consciousness does not give rise to materiality and materiality does
not give rise to consciousness. Moreover, there is no element of
"mindstuff" that is transmitted from one lifetime to the next. The
various states of existence that one takes in different lifetimes are
determined by the actions (*karma*) one has created in past lifetimes.
Insofar as actions proceed from the mental awareness, it can be said
that these various existences and constructions of self depend on
awareness. For this reason, the cultivation of mindfulness and awareness is critical.

With the exception of some Western converts, most Buddhists assume that life exists after death, though not in the form of a soul. An individual's previous identity falls away as the physical elements disintegrate and an impermanent stream of consciousness continues to a new rebirth. The next state of existence, or rebirth, will be in a pleasant or unpleasant realm, depending on the actions one has created over the course of many lifetimes. The most fortunate state of all is liberation, which frees one from further rebirth. In the Mahāyāna tradition, there is also the possibility of taking rebirth in a Pure Land, an extremely fortunate realm where Dharma teachings are given constantly, there are no distractions, and conditions are therefore highly conducive to achieving a state of perfect awakening, or Buddhahood (samyaksambuddha).

Differences of opinion about the nature of the transition from one lifetime to the next are found in different Buddhist cultures. Whereas Buddhists in Theravāda countries (Burma, Cambodia, Laos, Sri Lanka, and Thailand) most often believe that a person takes rebirth immediately after death, those in Mahāyāna countries (China, Japan, Korea, Mongolia, Taiwan, and Tibet) generally assume the possibility of a period of transition between death in one lifetime and rebirth in the next. In Tibet, this transitional period is known as the "intermediate state" (bardo) between death and rebirth or, more accurately, between death and re-conception. A large body of literature and wealth of religious practices developed around the idea of an intermediate state, including the well-known text popularly known as the Tibetan Book of the Dead.[6] As with most other aspects of Tibetan Buddhist belief and practice, the concept of an intermediate state can be traced to India and is integrally linked with Buddhist understandings of consciousness, personal identity, and the process of dying. An analysis of these fundamental and closely interwoven concepts provides the vocabulary for discussing Buddhist ideas about the experiences that may occur during the interval between one lifetime and the next. This discussion, in turn, provides a framework for considering Buddhist approaches to bioethical dilemmas.

Like most Buddhists, the seventh-century Indian philosopher Dharmakīrti assumes that a stream of mental moments continues uninterruptedly from one lifetime to the next. To verify the uninterrupted continuity of mental moments in the transitional state (bardo) through direct experience requires direct yogic perception (svasaṃvedana-pratyakṣha), which is attained through intensive meditation practice. But to verify the uninterrupted continuity of mental moments in the present lifetime requires only ordinary direct perception (pratyakṣha), which can be attained through simply sitting still and watching one's own thoughts. The nature of this uninterrupted stream of mental events (*citta*) is the subject matter of meditations on the nature of mind. In other words, although the mind is a rather illusive object of awareness at first, it is possible to verify the continuity of consciousness from one moment to the next through one's own direct experience. By watching the process by which one moment of mental awareness give rise to the next, moment to moment, it is possible to infer that an individual's stream of consciousness continues from this lifetime to the next. In this way, in the absence of evidence to the contrary, one can conclude through inferential valid cognition (*anumānaprāṇa*) that consciousness continues from one lifetime to the next. It is also believed that by watching the process of mental awareness in reverse during meditation, it is possible to verify the sequence of one's past rebirths through direct perception.

The presence of mental consciousness is the common denominator among all forms of sentient life and the crucial determinant of a sentient being. From a Buddhist point of view, the "certainty of self" that Freud refers to is no certainty at all, but rather the ultimate illusion. In Freud's view, pathology makes us aware that the boundary between oneself and the outside world is uncertain and contested.[7] Buddhists would concur with this, highlighting the uncertainty of this distinction by using the Four Foundations of Mindfulness (body, feelings, consciousness, and additional phenomena) as specific topics of analysis. Analysis is further focused on the question of when life begins, the demarcations between self and other-than-self, and the distinctions between life and death.

Although the notion of a soul, spirit, or enduring self is quite thoroughly refuted in Buddhist philosophical thought, that has not prevented divergent points of view from persisting in the popular mind. For example, Buddhists in East Asia commonly refer to the spirits of their loved ones as enduring beyond death and conduct ritual offerings to ensure their well-being in "the other world." Whether these beliefs and practices can be traced to Taoist origins or other traditions, a shrine room for offerings to the dead are found in many Buddhist temples and rituals are performed there everyday.[8] Especially when someone dies in a violent or unnatural way, as in an accident, a suicide, or a murder, ordinary Buddhists believe that the person's spirit is unhappy and wanders like a ghost—hungry, lonely, and dissatisfied. Chinese ghost stories are legendary, but similar beliefs are also found among Buddhists elsewhere, including Theravāda countries. In Cambodia, for example, Pchnum Benn is a two-week-long ceremony during which people offer rice and cakes to appease the unhappy spirits of nearly two million people who were tortured to death or died of starvation and disease under the Khmer Rouge. During Pol Pot's radical Maoist regime beginning in 1975, most of Cambodia's monks were murdered, so it was impossible to perform proper religious rites for the dead. Their tormented spirits are believed to still wander the countryside, so pagodas throughout the country sponsor these festivals at night, where the spirits of the dead, attracted by the scent of incense, congregate to partake of food offerings dedicated in their name.

The belief in souls and spirits are notable for many reasons. First, they dispel the myth that Buddhism is a monolith and the assumption that Buddhists speak with one voice about the nature of the self, consciousness, and the after-death state. Second, it reveals the enormous cultural diversity that can be found in the Buddhist world. Third, it points out the disparity that often exists between the views of scholars and philosophers, and the views of ordinary Buddhists in the temples. Fourth, it confirms that Buddhist teachings and practices are flexible and have transformed over time to meet the needs of people in vastly different circumstances. Because consciousness is subtle and its relationship to self-identity is complex, many different understandings of these topics are found in the Buddhist world. To understand more about how consciousness functions at death requires further analysis and reflection on the topic of self.

Chapter 4

Contemplating
Self and No-Self

A favorite theme of Buddhist contemplation is: "What is the self?" The inquiry is intimately related to death, because the construction of personal identity and its dissolution at the time of death are intrinsically related. If the self is not a living thing, but merely a concept or an abstraction, then how can it be subject to death? The intimate link between death and identity is a persistent topic of reflection in Buddhist thought, a topic of engagement on both the intellectual and experiential levels.

In reflecting on the self and death, Buddhist texts from both the Theravāda and Mahāyāna traditions analyze the components of the self in an effort to discover the true nature of the self. When one discovers that an independently existing self does not exist either among these components or apart from them, one concludes that the self does not exist as it appears to, but is simply a convenient label:

> In the *Milinda Pañha* [*The Questions of King Milinda*], when King Milinda asks a monk his name, the monk replies, "Sir, I am known as 'Nagasena'; my fellows in the religious life address me as 'Nagasena.' Although my parents gave (me) the name 'Nagasena' . . . it is just an appellation, a form of speech, a description, a conventional usage. 'Nagasena' is only a name, for no person is found here."[1]

In the *Milinda Pañha*, King Milinda further asks, "Who is reborn?" Nāgasena replies, "Name and form (*nāma-rūpa*)." "Name and form" is the fourth in a series of twelve "links" of dependent arising (*pratītya-samutpāda*) that explain the causal relationships that involve sentient beings in cyclic existence (*saṃsāra*).[2] Each of the twelve links of dependent arising functions as the condition for the arising of the next: ignorance (*avidyā*); mental formations (*saṃskāra*); consciousness (*vijñāna*); name and form (*nāma-rūpa*); the six senses (*ṣaḍāyatana*); contact (*sparśa*); feeling (*vedanā*); craving (*tṛṣṇā*); grasping (*upādāna*); becoming (*bhava*); birth (*jāti*); and aging and death (*jarāmaraṇa*). The point of this analysis is to understand how sentient beings become involved in cyclic existence and how they can reverse this chain of events. By overcoming ignorance, the first link of the chain, it is said that sentient beings can free themselves from the wheel of birth, death, and rebirth. Eliminating ignorance, particularly ignorance about the nature of the self, is therefore central to liberation from death, rebirth, and suffering.

Buddhists of all traditions reflect on the nature of self, using a variety of different methods. In the Korean Seon (Zen) tradition, for example, practitioners focus on the *koan* "What is it?" Specifically, they contemplate the question, "What is it that answers when someone calls your name?" In the Tibetan tradition, practitioners focus on the questions, "What is the I?" Intensive inquiry into the true nature of the self challenges familiar assumptions about the nature of the self that disintegrates at the time of death.

From a Buddhist perspective, reflections on the nature of the self are of central importance, because ignorance about the true nature of the self leads to many other problems. From ignorance arises an instinctual sense of self. On the basis of this instinctual sense of self, mistaken projections of "I," "me," and "mine" arise. On the basis of these mistaken projections, one misconceives other aspects of experience. The mistaken conception of the self as a fixed reality generates further misconceptions, conflicting emotions, and misguided actions. Understanding the self as a constructed reality helps to unravel fixed conceptions of reality and the meaning of life, death, happiness, and loss. Understanding death as a constructed reality raises further questions, especially about the extension and termination of life.

Identity and No-Self: Finding the Builder of the House

In the *Dhammapada* the Buddha is quoted as saying that freedom from rebirth is achieved through understanding the true nature of the self:

> I have gone through many rounds of birth and death, looking in vain for the builder of this body. Heavy indeed is birth and death again and again! But now I have seen you,

housebuilder, you shall not build this house again. Its beams are broken, its dome is shattered: self-will [grasping] is extinguished; *nirvāṇa* is attained.[3]

A false sense of a self arises from not paying close attention to the changes that occur in the body and mind every moment. Grasping at the false notion of self—the conceit of the "I"—is regarded as the root of all sufferings and dissatisfactions, and yet the attachment to self is so instinctual that one is often not even aware of it. An understanding of self and no-self is therefore critical for understanding how individuals move through life and what happens to them at the time of death.

Among the many Buddhist meditations that foster an understanding of the illusory nature of the self, one involves reflection on the different identities that sentient beings assume. For example, a single individual may assume several different identities—as a parent, a child, a teacher, a student, a lover, and a friend—even in the space of a day. Another meditation involves reflection on the shifting nature of identity over time. The image one sees in the mirror today is not the same image one saw yesterday, nor, regrettably, is it the same image that is reflected in a photograph from one's youth. One recognizes and identifies with the earlier image, yet it is very different from the image one sees reflected in the mirror and identifies with now. Another meditation involves reflection on the mutable nature of identity from one lifetime to the next. In the Buddhist worldview, sentient beings have been dying and taking rebirth within the various realms of cyclic existence (*saṃsāra*) since time without beginning. In this meditation, one contemplates on how individuals take birth in different genders, different classes of society, and different states of existence from lifetime to lifetime. All these reflections engender an awareness of the self as a mutable construct and challenge fixed notions of self.

The Buddhists surmise that the false construct of a self—the conceit of an "I"—is the root cause of the attachments and consequent disappointments living beings experience. One identifies with an image of the active, clever, attractive person one formerly was and feels dissatisfied that the image no longer matches reality. The more closely one identifies with the images from one's youth, the greater the unease and unhappiness one experiences when one no longer resembles those images. This unease increases with drastic changes, like illness, aging, and disabilities.

On a theoretical level, it is not difficult to understand that one's body and mind are changing from moment to moment, but psychologically one still clings to the timeless images one constructs. An investigation of the concepts of self and no-self is therefore a means to understand how human beings confuse the way things actually exist with the images they construct of things. From a Buddhist perspective, this deep-rooted misconception about the existence of a concrete and abiding self is common to all sentient beings. An investigation into the true versus the illusory nature of the self, through meditation, is therefore a direct application of the Buddha's injunction to see things "as they are."

One of the most basic Buddhist meditations on self and no-self involves reflection on the physical and psychological constituents that comprise the self. The idea is to look closely, and to become aware of the compounded, contingent nature of the self. When one pays close attention, one notices that the physical and mental components of the self change from moment to moment, in relation to shifting circumstances. It is said that, in meditation, it is possible to become aware of these changes even on a molecular or atomic level.

Despite the fact that the components of the self undergo incessant change, it is natural to assume the existence of a concrete, enduring, independently existing self, based on an apparent continuity of body and mind. Yet, when one tries to find an independently existing self, one comes up empty-handed. Diligent investigation into the nature of the self is therefore useful for developing insight into some very basic misconceptions about the self. These insights lead to a fundamental reevaluation of the way one understands the world and one's place within it.

From a Buddhist perspective, the belief in an enduring self arises from ignorance. Human beings instinctively tend to identify with the body and mind, assume the continuity of body and mind, and become attached to them. Upon reflection, however, it becomes obvious that the components of the self have been changing ever since the moment of birth and continue to change constantly. As the baby becomes a child and then an adult, there is an apparent continuity, despite major changes at each stage of development. Through meditation, however, one becomes aware that the body and mind are in a constant state of flux, and that the elements comprising body and mind are arising and perishing from moment to moment. Out of ignorance, a solid sense of self develops instinctively, based on a mistaken perception of the constituent elements of the self as enduring. In the Buddhist view, however, the superimposition of a solid, enduring self on these changing constituent elements is a fundamental misconception. Based on this basic misconception, one constructs an ongoing series of self-identifications, and develops attachments and expectations based on these constructs. In this continual process of mistaken identification, one confuses construct and reality, thereby setting oneself up for many difficulties and frustrations.

This process of mistaken identification also applies to the way one views others. Again, based on ignorance, one constructs images of others that may have little relation to reality, develops attachments and expectations based on these fundamental misconceptions, and then becomes disappointed when others do not behave consistently with the images that have been unrealistically projected. In theory, one knows that things are constantly changing, but in reality one gets disappointed nonetheless when things do not stay the way one wishes. For example, one feels miserable when loved ones get old, sick, and die, because one hopes they will stay young, healthy, and alive. The sadness one feels when things change is based on the mistaken perception that things are enduring, although, in fact, they are not. When one pays attention, it becomes clear that responses to one's environment and to other people are directly related to the images and expectations one projects. The sadness and disappointment one feels are proportionate to the extent of one's attachments, which clearly involve an element of self-interest. Instead of a pure concern for the happiness and well-being of others, one's emotional attachments and responses are generally mixed with one's own desires and expectations. When others do not fulfill expectations, feelings of dissatisfaction, frustration, anger, or betrayal arise. All these expectations—expecting to get something in return, expecting things to remain the same, or expecting things to change—are based on mistaken identifications, ultimately rooted in ignorance. Understanding these psychological processes requires a deeper analysis of the nature of self.

Looking more deeply into the nature of the self, the practitioner posits that, for the self to have ontological status, it must exist either apart from or identical with its component parts. The basic components of the self are the five aggregates (skandhas): form (rūpa), feelings (vedanā), perceptions (saṃjñā), karmic formations (saṃskāra),[4] and consciousness (vijñāna). The five aggregates are then analyzed one by one to see whether a self can be found anywhere among them. In meditation, one analyzes each of the aggregates and whether any of them can be identified as the self. Beginning with the form aggregate, one contemplates each part of the body, from head to foot, investigating whether any part of the body is equivalent to a self. If a self cannot be found among the various parts of body, one proceeds to an investigation of the second aggregate, the feelings. One contemplates the different types of feelings—pleasant, unpleasant, and neutral—investigating whether any of these feelings is equivalent to a self. If a self cannot be

found among the feelings, one proceeds to an analysis of the perceptions, karmic formations, and consciousness, in turn.

It may be tempting to identify the fifth aggregate, consciousness,
with the self, but this gambit does not hold up under scrutiny. The
term consciousness (*vijñāna*), defined as knowing (*saṃvedana*) and
awareness (*jñāna*), refers to discrete, causally conditioned moments of
sensory or mental awareness. The term consciousness may also be
used to denote the momentary stream of consciousness, or series of
conscious events that arise and perish from moment to moment. Each
moment of consciousness conditions the next, and an appearance of
continuity arises on the basis of the causal connectedness of these
momentary conscious events. Each sentient being possesses consciousness and each stream of consciousness is individual. Since sentient
beings are said to be infinite in number, their streams of consciousness
can also be said to be infinite in number. Each stream of consciousness
is said to have continued since beginningless time and each has the
potential, through mental cultivation, to become purified or liberated
from mental defilements and conflicting emotions. These streams of
consciousness have no known source and at no point do these individual streams of consciousness merge together or unite with something greater. Under investigation, it becomes apparent that the self
cannot be identified with any single moment of consciousness, nor
with the sum of these fleeting moments. The fifth aggregate, consciousness, is therefore not equivalent to a self.

Through this process of continuous, rigorous examination, the
practitioner sets out to understand the nature of the self and the relationship between body, consciousness, and self. It rapidly becomes
apparent that the self does not exist as it appears. The process of
investigation is a means of understanding how the elements of the self
arise in relation to causes and conditions, and therefore ultimately
lack any autonomous core. Eventually, one ascertains that the self
does not exist as any one of the five aggregates. Nor does the self exist
as the sum total of the aggregates, since the self would be diminished
when any of the aggregates could not be apprehended. Tibetan com-
mentators conclude that the self is not the combination of its component parts, but merely a label "imputed upon the basis of designation"
(Tib: *rtag pa btags dzam*). This conclusion follows from a certain logical
impasse: If one contends that the person is the total combination of
particular physical and mental component parts, then how many of
the parts can be subtracted before the person ceases to exist?

If a self cannot be located among the five aggregates through the
process of rigorous analysis, the next step is to investigate whether a

self exists apart from the aggregates. For a self to exist apart from the aggregates, it must be findable and the relationship between the self and the aggregates must be clear. Despite a thorough investigation, however, a self that exists apart from the aggregates cannot be found. Through this process of analytical contemplation, the practitioner comes to the conclusion that an independently existent self does not exist either among the constituent aggregates or apart from them. Because an independently existent self is nowhere to be found, the five aggregates are regarded as simply "the basis of imputation of a self," The notion of a self is therefore understood to be a convenient fiction for everyday functioning—something "merely imputed by terms and concepts."

To gain insight into the basic misconception of the self is not to deny the existence of the self altogether. The everyday self continues to function on a conventional level; the point is that this conventionally existent self lacks ultimate reality. Notions of individual identity are typically constructed on the basis of temporary markers, such as name, form, social status, and so on. When these impermanent markers change, one's sense of identity and view of the world also change, giving rise to feelings of uncertainty and anxiety. Intellectually, one can recognize that the physical and mental constituents of individual identity are temporary, changing from moment to moment. Yet out of ignorance, due to habitual misconceptions, one still instinctively assumes that the self is enduring and grasps at the illusion of a solid self as being real. On the basis of a fundamental misconception about the nature of the self, a host of further misconceptions, dissatisfactions, and disappointments arises. When things do not match one's expectations, one feels frustrated, disconcerted, or discouraged. For Buddhists, liberation means to become free from the basic misconception of the self and the afflictive emotions that result from that misconception.

The Buddhist concept of no-self is frequently misunderstood as being nihilistic. From a Buddhist perspective, however, the theory of no-self does not negate the conventional self, nor does it negate the possibility of rebirth.[5] The continuity of causal connectedness—between moments of consciousness, actions (*karma*), and the effects of actions— is insufficient grounds for asserting the existence of an enduring self, but this does not nullify the self altogether. No Buddhist school denies that the constructed self exists and functions on a conventional level, even though it lacks ultimate existence. There is no attempt to do away with the reflexive pronoun; in fact, the texts include frequent ethical and religious injunctions to purify oneself, guard oneself, search for oneself, be an island unto oneself, be the lord of oneself, to reproach oneself, and so on. What is denied is the existence of the self as an independently existing and enduring reality, not the conventional self. As Steven Collins puts it, an enlightened individual no longer has a sense of "I" and is not led astray by the use of the first person.[6]

The Buddha refuted the extremes of both nihilism and eternalism. The view of absolute nonexistence (*nāstivāda*) is untenable, because it contradicts one's own direct experience of phenomenal reality. The view of absolute existence (*astivāda*) is also untenable, because it contradicts one's direct experience of things disintegrating. Instead, the Buddha is said to have asserted a middle ground between the two extremes: phenomena exist conventionally, but not ultimately. The fact that human beings see and name things is evidence that things exist on some level, but the ability to see and name things does not mean that they exist on an essential or absolute level. By the same token, to deny the true existence of the self is not to deny the existence of the self altogether. The self is said to be illusory by nature, but this does not mean that the self is merely an illusion or totally nonexistent. It simply means that the self does not exist as it appears to exist and is therefore illusory in appearance. A careful distinction must therefore be made between the assertions that: (1) the self does not exist ultimately, and (2) the self ultimately does not exist. The first statement correctly asserts that there is no ultimate existence to the self; the second incorrectly states that the self ultimately does not exist at all.

Grasping (*upādāna*) is the ninth of the twelve links of dependent arising that keep sentient beings cycling in the wheel of repeated rebirth. The four types of grasping are: (1) grasping at sense pleasures, (2) grasping at rules and rituals, (3) grasping at views, and (4) grasping at the idea of an independently existing self. Grasping at the self as independently existing is the most fundamental type of grasping, because it leads directly to the following links: existence, birth, and aging and death. A liberated being (*arhat*) is one who has developed direct insight into the true nature of the self and has therefore become free from greed, hatred, attachment, jealousy, pride, and all the other afflictive emotions that arise from grasping at the self. For this reason, to eradicate grasping at the self is regarded as crucial for achieving liberation from cyclic existence.

The Paradox of the Self: Evolving Interpretations

The Buddha's theory of no-self (*anātman*) was apparently a response to earlier Indian beliefs and directly contradicted two fundamental philosophical assumptions: the existence of an unchanging ultimate reality (Brahman) and an unchanging self (*ātman*). The concept of no-self was not readily understandable, though, and was often misinterpreted as nihilistic. Some even contend that the Buddha avoided a categorical denial of self, sensing that the topic would lead to endless speculation and disputes. And, indeed, the concept of *anātman* has continued to be the subject of ongoing debate, even among the Buddhists, for hundreds of years. Some 200 years after the Buddha's passing, for example, a teacher by the name of Vātsīputra propounded the existence of a person that exists apart from the five aggregates, giving rise to the Pudgalavāda (Personalist) School. This view never gained wide acceptance, however, and there is a general scholarly consensus, based on numerous scriptural references, that the Buddha denied the existence of a self apart from its constituent elements. For example, when asked to explain the phrase "the world is empty," the Buddha explains that it means the world is "empty of self and what belongs to self."[7]

The Buddhist theory of no-self has been persistently critiqued by Indian philosophers of other schools up to the present day. The recurrent questions are: Without a self, who experiences the results of virtuous and non-virtuous deeds? If there is no self, what travels from life to life? The Buddhists respond to these questions by asserting that the ripening of *karma* does not require the existence of an *ātman*. Just as the flame from one candle lights another candle without anything passing between them, the imprints of actions influence successive moments of consciousness without anything substantial passing between them. The skillful or unskillful actions created in one lifetime give rise to pleasant or unpleasant circumstances in the future, in accordance with the law of cause and effect, but the process is by no means contingent upon an independently existent self. The *Tattvasaṃgraha* is one of many texts that respond in detail to the claim that the no-self doctrine is inadequate to account for *karma* and rebirth. The text argues that the doctrine of self is no more adequate than the theory of no-self to explain the apparent continuity of persons and phenomena from one moment to the next.

In the basic teachings found in the early Pāli texts and further elaborated in the Mahāyāna literature, the self designates the composite of constantly changing physical and mental components of the self that arise in dependence on causes and conditions. As in the Pāli canon, the Mahāyāna texts explain that mistakenly conceiving the self to be independently existent and enduring is the source of many afflictive mental states and unskillful actions. These texts further explain how, by developing insight into the true nature of the self, an individual can eradicate attachment to the self, progress through the paths and stages of realization, and eventually achieve enlightenment.

The paradox of the *arhat* achieving liberation for himself or herself through insight into no-self is apparent even in the earliest Buddhist texts. This paradox is accentuated in the Prajñāpāramitā literature of the Mahāyāna tradition, where the *bodhisattva* strives for enlightenment for himself or herself, while simultaneously eradicating attachment to self. The concept of *prajñā*, the wisdom that understands the empty (*śūnya*) nature of all phenomena becomes key in understanding the paradoxical nature of the self, which exists conventionally but not ultimately. In the Mahāyāna tradition, the goal is to become a perfectly awakened Buddha, and this goal is thought to be desirable and attainable by all sentient beings, each of whom individually achieves enlightenment. There are three prerequisites for entering the path to Buddhahood: renunciation (of *saṃsāra*), *bodhicitta* (the enlightened attitude of wishing to achieve perfect awakening in order to liberate all beings from suffering), and direct insight into emptiness (*śūnyatā*). Although interpretations of emptiness differ from school to school, the ultimately non-dual nature of *saṃsāra* and *nirvāṇa*, of conventional and ultimate reality, is central to all schools of Mahāyāna thought, influencing Mahāyāna perspectives on death and identity in India and the philosophical systems that evolved in Tibet and East Asia.

The Mahāyāna texts specifically explain that the theory of no-self applies not only to persons, but to all other phenomena as well. In this view, the three characteristics of existence—unsatisfactoriness (*duhkha*), impermanence (*anitya*), and no-self (*anātman*)—apply to all conditioned things equally. As in ealier Buddhist schools, insight into these three is the gateway to higher attainments. Like the self, other phenomena also exist as conventional realities, but lack any core reality. In a well-known analogy, the nun Vajīra asks: "What is the cart?" "Is it the axle? Or the wheels, or the chassis, or reins, or yoke that is the chariot? Is it all of these combined, or is it something apart from them?"[8] Questioning in this way, practitioners analyze phenomena into their component parts in an effort to discover their true nature. This analysis is even applied to non-existent phenomena, which are also characterized as lacking self.

Tibetan scholars analyze the self in accordance with the Mahāyāna doctrine of the two truths. The self is a functional phenomenon that, like all phenomena, exists on the level of conventional truth (*saṃvṛtisatya*), but does not exist on the level of ultimate truth (*paramārtha-satya*). This theory of two levels of truth is used to explain the apparent continuity of phenomenal events and the simultaneous lack of true existence of self and phenomena. The conventional and ultimate levels of truth are mutually entailing; that is to say, all conditioned things are empty of true existence and each thing has its specific emptiness. The classic example is a vase and the emptiness of the vase. The vase is characterized as empty (*śūnya*), because it is empty of true existence. The conventional truth of the vase is its everyday functional existence; the ultimate truth of the vase is its emptiness—the fact that it lacks true existence. The ultimate truth of the vase—the emptiness of the vase—therefore exists in dependence on the conventional existence of the vase. When the vase shatters, the emptiness of the vase also comes to an end.[9] In this way, dependent arising (*pratītya-samutpāda*) and emptiness are understood to be mutually entailing. As the *Sāgaramatiparipṛchchhā* says: "Those which arise dependently are free of inherent existence."[10] As the Madhyamaka master Nāgārjuna (2nd–3rd century) states in the *Treatise on the Middle Way*:

> That which arises dependently
> We explain as emptiness.
> That [emptiness] is dependent designation;
> Just it is the middle path.

> Because there is no phenomenon
> That is not a dependent-arising,
> There is no phenomenon
> That is not empty.[11]

In other words, phenomena are empty of true existence because they arise dependently and phenomena arise dependently because they are empty of true existence. If things existed independently or ultimately, they would be impervious to change, and evolution would be impossible, but there is no verifiable evidence of such an independent reality.

In the Mahāyāna Buddhist schools, the concept of self is also discussed in terms of self-cherishing and self-grasping. Self-cherishing denotes cherishing oneself more than others; self-grasping denotes grasping at oneself as being truly existent. Each of these mistaken attitudes needs to be understood and eventually eliminated, by applying both conventional and ultimate antidotes. The conventional antidotes to self-cherishing are loving kindness and compassion—cherishing others more than oneself. The ultimate antidote to self-cherishing is *bodhicitta*, the enlightened attitude of wishing to achieve the state of perfect Buddhahood in order to liberate all sentient beings from suffering. The conventional antidote to self-grasping is meditation on impermanence—realizing the fragile, fleeting nature of one's own existence. The ultimate antidote to self-grasping is the wisdom (*prajñā*) that directly understands emptiness (*śūnyatā*). This wisdom is an awareness of things "as they are," without such false projections such as "I," "me," and "mine."

Developing wisdom (*prajñā*) is key to understanding how the self is mistakenly perceived by ordinary beings. First, the self is mistakenly perceived to be independently existent, when in fact it exists in dependence on the five aggregates.[12] Second, the self is mistakenly perceived to be enduring, when in fact it is impermanent. Third, the self is mistakenly perceived to exist truly, when in fact it is merely imputed to exist based on its constituent parts. This imputed existence (*prajñaptisat*) is then misinterpreted as true existence.[13] To eradicate ignorance or "unknowing" (*avidyā*), the root of all other delusions, is to eliminate the misconception of the self as existing independently of its bases of imputation. When ignorance is eradicated, the first link in the chain of dependent arising that traps sentient beings in *saṃsāra* is eliminated. Nāgārjuna expresses it this way:

> Having seen thus the aggregates as untrue,
> The conception of I is abandoned,
> And due to abandoning the conception of I
> The aggregates arise no more.[14]

When the self and the aggregates are no longer conceived as being truly existent, the afflictive emotions and unwholesome actions based on these misconceptions are eliminated. When unwholesome actions no longer create the causes of suffering, liberation from suffering is attained. Without attachment to self, there is nothing to which suffering can adhere.

Direct insight into emptiness is taught as the perfect antidote for ignorance, particularly the fundamental ignorance that grasps at the notion of self. In response to the canonical statement, "In liberation there is no self and no aggregates," Nāgārjuna says that to mistake the illusory self for a true self is as foolish as to mistake a mirage for water.[15] For Nāgārjuna, to understand the true nature of the self is no mere abstraction, but is directly relevant to issues of death and liberation. For example, he says, "If we are not afraid of the termination of self that comes with liberation, why do we fear the termination of the self at death?"[16]

The Buddhist literature that was transmitted to Tibet includes extensive discussions about the nature of the self, and how the basic misconception of an enduring self leads to problems in an impermanent world. Misconceptions about the self are among the three fundamental misconceptions that lie at the root of all afflictions. These three are: conceiving what is impermanent as permanent, what is undesirable as desirable, and what is lacking self as having self. Clinging to the misconception of a self, whether consciously or unconsciously, conceptually or instinctively, is integrally linked with grasping at permanence, and grasping at permanence is a source of suffering. Because human beings mistakenly perceive conditioned things (bodies, minds, possessions, achievements, and so on) to be enduring, they become confused and unhappy when things fall apart. All illusions of permanence are shattered most starkly when human beings face serious illness and death, and the chimera of a solid self begins to shatter. Because they strongly identify with the self and carry on as if it truly existed, the approach of death and the impending loss of the self can be a source of misery and bewilderment.

To summarize, the concept of no-self (*anātman*) is central to Buddhist metaphysics and integrally related to the theories of *karma*, rebirth, and liberation. The "self" is simply a convenient designation for a combination of mental and physical components that are ultimately devoid of any essence, soul, or independent identity. An essentialized notion of self is refuted, for three reasons. First, by definition, an essentialized self would be static, immutable, and impervious to change and evolution, whereas change is observable in everyday experience. Second, an essentialized self would be unaffected by social, political, and environmental factors, whereas ordinary beings are strongly affected by these factors. Third, an essentialized self would be uncaused, whereas in the Buddhist view all conditioned things arise in dependence on causes and conditions. The Buddhists therefore reject a concretized, reified concept of self, positing instead a contingent, contextual, interdependent concept of self. This refutation of a fixed self is central to Buddhist psychology and ethics.

Understanding the self as a constructed and constantly changing phenomenon (the "right view") not only avoids the extremes of nihilism and eternalism, but is also the key to higher realizations and liberation. An understanding of no-self helps counteract feelings of attachment, pride, and anger that arise as a result of misconceiving the conventional self to be truly existent. Meditations on death, impermanence, and no-self help to counteract fixed notions of self, beginning at a gross material level and eventually leading to a realization of the contingent nature of the self. Continuous intensive contemplation gradually counteracts attachment to even the most subtle sense of self. Contemplation on no-self is thus thought to be the best all-round antidote to reified notions of self and world, and to the problems that arise from these mistaken notions.

Death and Disintegration

Through contemplation—alternating theoretical analysis and meditative stabilization on the absence of a substantial self that exists either
among or apart from the aggregates—one gains insight into the true
nature of the self as illusory. With this insight the next question is
how, in the absence of an independently existent self, actions (karma)
produce consequences in this and future lifetimes.[17] If there is no soul
or self underlying successive discrete moments of consciousness, it is
necessary to explain how actions created in one lifetime give rise to
pleasant or unpleasant consequences in future lifetimes. If the body
and other aggregates disintegrate at the time of death, who experiences rebirth and the results of actions created in the past? With no
independent soul or locus of individual identity, how can the rebirth
linkage be explained? What becomes of the conventional self at the
time of death and what, if anything, continues?

Buddhist theories of self, karma, dependent arising, and ethics
are closely interwoven. Ignorance is the first link in the chain of dependent arising that explains how sentient beings become involved in
cyclic existence in the first place. Due to ignorance, especially ignorance about the true nature of the self, a host of afflictive emotions
arise that enmesh sentient beings in unwholesome actions that lead to
further rebirth. With intelligence, however, this process can be re-
versed. Because human beings are capable of logical reasoning and
have the freedom to make ethical decisions, they have the potential to
extricate themselves from the cycle by understanding how ignorance,
attachment to self, and mental defilements act as its root causes. Other
living beings, such as the animals, also have bodies, minds, needs,
desires, and their own personal histories, but these attributes alone are
insufficient for ethical decision making. For this reason, human beings' potential for liberation is regarded as far greater than that of the
animals and other sentient beings. Diligent practitioners may achieve
liberation within just a few lifetimes.

In the Brahmanical view that prevailed at the Buddha's time, the
concept of rebirth made sense only if there were an enduring ātman
(self) that reincarnated from lifetime to lifetime, taking on a new body
each time. Broadly speaking, these and other non-Buddhist theories
about what happens to an individual at death reduce to: (1) there
exists a fundamental core of being (soul, self, ātman), beyond the physical components that undergo change, (2) the self is replaced by something entirely different at death, or (3) the self disappears at death.
The Buddhist theory of a momentary, insubstantial self contrasts with

and is persistently critiqued by proponents of these other theories. For example, proponents of an *ātman* critique the concept of no-self as being inadequate to sustain a cogent ethical theory. The Buddhists attempt to refute these opposing positions, using a variety of arguments. The analogy of a flame from one candle that lights another, as mentioned earlier, is used to explain how consciousness is rekindled in a future life, without anything substantial passing from one existence to the next. Various other analogies are used to explain how *karma* ripens, that is, how the consequences of actions are experienced in the absence of a substantial self. The theories of *karma*, self, and rebirth are all being reevaluated in current discussions of applied ethics, especially as Buddhism spreads to new cultural contexts and confronts a wide range of new questions and challenges.

The Buddhist theories of self and no-self are relevant to discussions of death and dying, because all constructed identities come to an end at the time of death. The more strongly one identifies with the fabricated self, the more difficult it will be to accept one's dissolution and death. Human beings feel at home in the body, take care of it, defend it from dangers, and protect it from the elements and illnesses. Because of this long-standing association with the body, it is understandable that the signs of aging and personal disintegration are a source of misery. The process of aging may be a teacher for a seasoned practitioner, but for the ordinary person without direct insight into the impermanent, constructed nature of the self, distress is inevitable when the hair turns white, teeth fall out, digestion fails, and memory starts to fade. Insight into the contingent, illusory nature of personal identity is useful when the body and mind begin to deteriorate, because without this awareness, the dissolution of the elements of the self at the time of death may come as an unpleasant shock and disrupt the process of a smooth transition from one life to the next.

There is no question that death is the end of life as we know it. That being the case, from a Buddhist perspective, it is essential to prepare for the end of life through mental cultivation (*bhāvana*) to ensure a propitious transition to the next state of existence. Over many centuries, Buddhist scholars and practitioners have discussed and reflected on the process of transitting from one existence to another. Some have also wondered whether the nature of this passage is worthy of speculation, contending that attention should be focused fully on the present moment instead. In any case, although the exact nature of the transition from one state of existence to the next is subject to debate, Buddhists concur that the identity of the conventional self comes to an end at the time of death. All that matters at that point is the actions one has created and the quality of one's mental cultivation. The end of the conventional self may not be the end of the story, however.

Tibetan scholars certainly found the end of life, the afterlife, and the idea of a transitional phase from one life to another worthy of speculation. Numerous literary works in Tibetan pertain to death and the intermediate state between death and re-conception, known as the *bardo*. This literature includes meditations on death and an elaborate technology for negotiating the states of the dying process, including advice on how to cope with fear, uncertainty, and a range of sensory and visionary experience. The guidance offered in manuals such as the so-called *Tibetan Book of the Dead* (*Bardo Tödrol*) is quite specific. It counsels the intermediate being to be aware of its immaterial state and to see all apparitions as mental constructs. There is no longer any need to fear death, because the person is already clinically dead. Relieved of the fear of impending death, the consciousness is free to rest in its own true nature. The goal is to maintain mental calm and clarity throughout the process of dying and to understand all the phenomena of the mind as mere appearances. In this way, ideally it will be possible to achieve realization and liberation, or at least an optimal rebirth.

For the experienced meditator, dying is an opportunity to collect the subtle energies or "winds" of the body into the central psychic channel at the heart center (*anāhata-chakra*), and to either attain liberation or direct the consciousness to a favorable rebirth.[18] For the untrained individual, however, death can be a frightening prospect. The ordinary consciousness, accustomed only to distracted, unproductive, and unwholesome thoughts, is unable to rest in the quietude of its own true nature or to direct itself to a fortunate state of rebirth. Anxious and confused, the untrained mind runs amok at the time of death, thereby forfeiting an opportunity for awakening. Instead of transiting calmly to the next state of existence, the mind becomes helpless before its own fears and karmic propensities, creating the causes of an unfortunate rebirth.

In contemporary discourse, the term "subject" is often used to denote the self, but in Buddhist usage the term subject is closer to the definition of consciousness, that is, the subject of valid cognition, or simply the knowing of phenomena. "Knowing and awareness" is a classic Buddhist definition of consciousness. Knowing and awareness are momentary by nature and no "knower," or subject of the knowing analogous to a substantial self, is implied.

According to the various Buddhist schools, consciousness does not simply cease at death, but continues to give rise to subsequent moments of consciousness in another state of existence. There are five types of sensory awareness or sense consciousness: visual, auditory, olfactory, gustatory, and tactile consciousness. These five types of consciousness arise from contact between the sense faculties and their respective physical objects: visual forms, sounds, smells, tastes, and physical sensations. Mental consciousness arises from contact between the mental faculty and an object of mental consciousness, such as an mental image, memory, or idea. In contrast to the five types of sense consciousness, mental consciousness may be present even in the absence of the body, as mentioned above in regard to beings of the formless realm.

Because consciousness is the center of all experience and the faculty that enables individuals to reflect on life and death, it is tempting to equate consciousness with a self or soul. If consciousness were permanent and enduring, this might be the case. But in the Buddhist analysis of consciousness, there is nothing permanent and enduring about consciousness at all. Just by sitting in silence and watching the mind, one quickly gains insight into the fleeting, ephemeral nature of consciousness, which is changing every moment. By verifying the impermanent nature of consciousness through direct personal experience in this way, it becomes obvious that consciousness is too changeable to constitute an enduring self. From this insight into the fleeting nature of consciousness, one begins to understand that there is no permanence to consciousness or to the self.

Because consciousness is the center of all experience, it may be assumed that cognitive death is the death of the person. Cognition is not the only function of consciousness, however. Conscious awareness may also be non-conceptual. For example, when someone smells a flower or a brownie, there is a moment of direct perception or awareness that occurs before the cognitive faculties of the mind begin to identify, label, and evaluate that perception. Furthermore, consciousness is present during dreamless sleep or when one is unconscious, even in the absence of cognitive thought. For these reasons, it is not at all certain that the cessation of cognitive functioning is the end of one's conscious experiences. If consciousness continues after the death of the body, the commonly accepted view that a person dies when the brain dies does not necessarily hold. In that case, the cessation of respiration, cardiac function, and brain function would be inadequate determinants of death. Death is ordinarily juxtaposed to life, such that the cessation of the vital signs are taken to indicate death. If consciousness continues after the cessation of the vital signs, however, then the deceased cannot conclusively be said to be dead.

If consciousness continues, then the experiences of a person in the process of dying are not solely dependent on the presence or absence of the physical body. Although the continuity of consciousness after death cannot be scientifically verified at present, it is not impossible that the technologies necessary to verify the presence or absence of consciousness may be developed at some future time. Meanwhile, most Buddhists assume that consciousness continues after clinical death, in an extremely subtle form, and the remainder prefer to leave the question open.

From a Buddhist perspective, conditioned things are said to exist by virtue of being the object of a valid cognition by a perceiving consciousness. In the Buddhist lexicon, a person may be said to exist based on a valid cognition of one or more of the five aggregates. A valid cognition does not require that all five aggregates be perceived; the existence of a person can be inferred simply by hearing the person's voice or seeing the person's form. To take another example, a being in a formless state of existence is said to exist solely by virtue of possessing consciousness. From these examples, a Buddhist may conclude that sentient beings do not cease to exist when the body disintegrates, as long as consciousness continues. Based on the presence of consciousness alone, it is possible that some sort of incipient being continues after death, even without any soul or enduring self.

The subtle continuity of mental consciousness, sometimes called the re-linking consciousness, is not identified with any specific form or realm of rebirth, human or otherwise. Sentient beings take different forms in different states of existence over many lifetimes, in accordance with their particular *karma* and level of mental development. Animals and other sentient beings all undergo this process of cyclic existence, but only human beings have the intelligence to recognize it and do something about it.

Understanding the different identities sentient beings assume in the incessant process of rebirth—female and male, human and animal, of different shapes and colors—decreases one's strong attachment to self-identity. Although there is a constructed self that evolves in relation to social and cultural context, the notion of self is not simply a theoretical abstraction or cultural construct. The innate grasping at self is what spontaneously arises and feels threatened when one is falsely accused or physically attacked. This innate sense of self is much more subtle, intimate, and deeply ingrained than the constructed self, having been constantly reinforced through innumerable lifetimes. The cherished illusion of the self is not merely an habitual mode of perception; it is also the essential pivot of all personal projects, social interactions, and perceptions. This innate sense of an essentialized self ignores the fleeting, contextual nature of human experience. Insight into the true nature of the self therefore allows one to stop grasping at the self and begin to make decisions within a larger ethical frame-work. To see beyond self is therefore to see beyond self-interest and ultimately to move beyond birth and death.

Chapter 5

Foundations of Buddhist Ethics

Buddhist texts from different places and periods present a variety of responses to questions about the nature of self, the nature of death, and what transpires in the process of a person's dying. For Buddhist practitioners, there is also an active engagement with death in meditation. Formulas like "The only thing that separates us from death is one breath," and "There is no guarantee which will come first, tomorrow or the next life," are constant reminders of the impermanent nature of human existence, enjoining practitioners to live each moment as if it were their last. The breath, the gossamer link between life and death, is a favorite mnemonic in Buddhist mindfulness practice. The rising and falling of the breath mirrors the arising and perishing of each moment—a continual reminder that living beings begin dying the moment they are born.

Buddhist texts describe analytical and experiential meditations on death, and especially recommend practice in cemeteries. To gain insight into death and impermanence, the practitioner reflects upon the fact that all compounded phenomena invariably disintegrate, all that is born must die. A standard meditation on death begins by contemplating that all living beings inevitably must die, the time of death is unpredictable, and at the time of death only one's spiritual practice, good deeds, and mental cultivation will be of any value. Possessions, loved ones, and worldly accomplishments will be of no use and may even become an impediment at the moment of death, if anger, fear, or attachment arises. Preparing for death by cultivating the mind will help one face death peacefully and mindfully, while the virtuous actions created throughout one's life will be the causes for a positive rebirth.

Contemplation on death helps us gain realization of the finitude and fragility of the body, helps dispel the illusion of our individuality and specialness, and motivates us to strive for liberation. Among the advantages of meditation on death and impermanence is that this awareness cuts through sensual desire, desire for rebirth, ignorance, and the conceit of the "I." Because death deprives us the objects of our attachment, meditation is useful for cutting through these attachments. The primary benefit of meditation on death is that it motivates us to practice diligently.

The *Visuddhimagga*, a fifth-century text by Buddhaghosa, explains many methods of contemplating death.[1] For example, the eight recollections on death include reflections on: (1) coming face-to-face with death as the executioner; (2) the loss of prosperity; (3) the inevitable lot of all living beings; (4) the countless factors, internal and external, that can cause death[2]; (5) the imminence of death; (6) the uncertainty of the time of death; (7) the definite limits of the life span; and (8) the brevity of each moment that brings one closer to death. The meditation on a rotting corpse, one of the thirteen *dutangas* (austerities) designed to generate renunciation, is even more graphic. It involves visiting a charnel ground daily to observe and reflect on the stages of decomposition of corpses. One reflects on the ten impurities of the rotting corpse as: (1) swollen, (2) discolored, (3) festering, (4) fissured, (5) mangled, (6) dismembered, (7) cut, (8) bloody, (9) worm-infested, and (10) skeletal.[3] These meditations make it impossible to deny the reality of death and spur one to prepare for death through intensive practice.

Buddhist Definitions of Life and Death

In the early Indian Buddhist scheme of things, the principle of nonharm (*ahiṃsa*), to avoid causing death or injury to sentient life, was a supreme value. Each living being had its own allotted life span as a result of its own karma and a death that occurred as a result of an accident was regarded as untimely, though accidents are regarded as the result of karma, too. Buddhaghosa explains this distinction in his commentary on mindfulness of death:

> Herein, *death* (*maraṇa*) is the interruption of the life faculty included within a single becoming (existence). . . . As intended here it is of two kinds, that is to say, timely death and untimely death. Herein, *timely death* comes about with the exhaustion of merit or with the exhaustion of a life span or with both. *Untimely death* comes about through kamma that interrupts kamma.[4]

In the case of a timely death, the life span is allowed to run its natural course until that person's store of merit is exhausted; an untimely death is one that occurs before that.

According to the Saṃyutta Nikāya and Majjhima Nikāya, death occurs when the vitality, heat, and consciousness leave the body.[5] Of these three, it is possible to measure the vitality and heat as indicated by the vital signs, but there is as yet no way to clinically measure consciousness or to determine the precise moment that the consciousness departs from the body. The Majjhima Nikāya explains that a person's conscious faculties depend upon vitality, and that vitality and heat are mutually interdependent, like light and a flame. However, later texts state that consciousness can exist even in the absence of heat and vitality, for example, the consciousness of a being in the intermediate state between death and re-conception or the consciousness of beings in the formless realm.[6] For Buddhists, the idea that consciousness continues after death is not unreasonable. After all, the stream of consciousness continues during sleep and even when one falls unconscious, so it is also possible that consciousness in some subtle form continues after the heartbeat and respiration wane. Even if one's conscious faculties, such as memory and discrimination, are dependent upon the life force and decline as heat and vitality ebb from the body, this does not negate the existence of a subtle continuum of mental consciousness.

If this is the case, the subtle consciousness may be present even in the absence of any gross conscious functions or physical signs of life such as breathing and pulse. An individual in a state of deep sleep or trance is not consciously aware, but is not devoid of consciousness. Some subtle consciousness must be present or the person would be dead. From a Buddhist point of view, it is not necessary for a person to be alive for consciousness to continue. Even though the presence of consciousness may not be clinically verifiable, the subtle consciousness may be present. It is unclear whether a person who is kept alive artificially necessarily possesses consciousness. Death is indicated when a person's gross conscious functions decline and will not revive, but even in the absence of brain function, a person's subtle mental consciousness may continue. The presence of the subtle consciousness is indicated by warmth in the body, generally observable in the area of the heart, whereas the absence of warmth in the area of the heart indicates death. When the subtle consciousness leaves the body, this warmth disappears and the person is dead. From a Tibetan Buddhist perspective, the signal that death has occurred is when the body begins to decompose and give off a disagreeable odor. When the body is artificially kept alive, however, questions arise about whether traditional indicators of death apply.

The Tibetan medical system, which derives from India, is predicated upon the three humors: wind, bile, and phlegm. Of the five winds (Skt. *prāna*, Tib. *srog rlung*) that are necessary for living a healthy life, it is the life-sustaining wind (Tib. *srog rlung*) that is specifically responsible for maintaining life.[7] This wind corresponds to the life faculty (Skt. *jīvaindriya*) or life force, which is equivalent to vitality (Skt. *ayus*). When the continuity of this life force is severed, death occurs. The presence of this wind is what determines whether a person is alive, but the presence of consciousness is what determines whether a person exists. This distinction is the demarcation between life and death in the Buddhist frame.

According to the 1968 Harvard definition, death is the absence of brain functions, specifically inactivity of the brain stem. Further research is needed to ascertain whether this definition is adequate to explain death from a Buddhist point of view. Buddhist texts, early or late, give no definition of death beyond that it is the cessation of vitality, respiration, and consciousness. The cessation of brain functions alone does not ensure that consciousness is no longer present, however. Although the functioning of the five sense faculties or powers (*indriya*) may depend on their respective physical sense organs (eye, ear, nose, tongue, and body), the functioning of mental consciousness is dependent on the mental faculty or power, which is not physical. Mental consciousness arises as a result of contact between the mental faculty and an object of cognition, not a physical sense organ. Because it is not dependent on the body, mental consciousness may continue in some form, despite the cessation of brain functions. The consciousness that continues after death is so subtle that most living beings are not consciously aware of it.

If atrophy of the cerebral cortex indicates that grosser levels of consciousness have ceased, it may also indicate the death of the individual, that is, the end of individual identity. But because the causal connectedness of the individual's consciousness may continue on to a new existence, from a Buddhist perspective, the atrophy of the cerebral cortex does not necessarily signal the end of the mental continuum. As long as the mental continuum is understood to be contingent and impermanent, it can be said to take another existence. But we cannot speak of the continuity of an individual, because after death that individual no longer exists. When the subtle mental consciousness continues to the next state of existence, it will take on another identity.

Emptiness in Early Buddhist Literature

In early Buddhist literature the term emptiness (*śūnyatā*) is used in at least three distinguishable ways. The first usage of the term indicates a mere absence. For example, renunciants (śrāmaṇa) are advised to meditate in empty places. The second usage also indicates an absence, specifically the absence of mental defilements. For example, greed, hatred, and delusion are said to be absent in the mind of a liberated being (arhat). The third usage signifies no-self, the lack of a substantial self among the five aggregates (skandhas). In the Saṃyutta Nikāya, in response to a query about the nature of the world, the Buddha explains, "Ānanda, as it is void of self or anything pertaining to self, therefore it is said, 'The world is void (Pāli: suñña).' "[8] The terms emptiness and no-self are often used interchangeably in the early Buddhist canon.[9]

In the Mahāyāna texts that began to appear in India around the first and second centuries CE, emptiness becomes a pivotal concept. For example, the Prajñāhṛdaya Sūtra (Heart of Wisdom Sūtra), perhaps the most popular of all Mahāyāna texts, explains that all phenomena are by nature empty, and uses the five skandhas as an example: "At that time, also, the great bodhisattva Avalokiteśvara saw the aspects of the profound and powerful perfection of wisdom and saw that the five aggregates are by nature empty."[10] The five skandhas are not the only things that are empty, however. In addition to a new emphasis on the bodhisattva concept, Mahāyāna texts draw a distinction between recognizing the emptiness of persons and the emptiness of phenomena. The concept of no-self is extended beyond persons to include all phenomena. Direct insight into emptiness, the lack of true existence of phenomena, is a quality attributed to the bodhisattva from the first stage (bhūmi) onward. The realization of emptiness is extolled as superior to the śrāvakas' "mere" realization of the selflessness of persons.

Distinguishing the Madhyamaka and Yogācāra Schools

The Mahāyāna tradition is distinguished from earlier schools of Buddhist thought and practice by advancing the ideal that all sentient beings can and should aspire to the perfect enlightenment of a Buddha. Toward this end, one aspires to become a bodhisattva. According to the Indian scholar and monk Atiśa, a bodhisattva is an individual who is characterized by renunciation, the altruistic aspiration to achieve perfect awakening in order to liberate all sentient beings from suffering (bodhicitta), and direct insight into emptiness (śūnyatā).[11] The bodhisattva ideal is the most prominent distinguishing characteristic of the Mahāyāna path. The concept of the bodhisattva occurs in the Pāli canon, but there it generally refers to the Buddha as he transversed the bodhisattva path in past lives on his way to Buddhahood. In the earlier, pre-Mahāyāna texts, the goal for most practitioners is to become an *arhat*. Because of the enormous difficulties of the pursuit, only exceptional individuals, such as Buddha Śākyamuni in a past life, aspire to become a fully awakened one (*samyaksambuddha*). In the Mahāyāna texts, to become a *bodhisattva* and eventually a fully awakened Buddha becomes the goal of all practitioners. In these texts, the qualities and attainments of a Buddha come to be regarded as vastly superior to those of an *arhat*.

Around the seventh century, two major schools gradually emerged from among the various streams of Mahāyāna thought in India: Madhyamaka and Yogācāra. According to Tibetan scholars, the Madhyamaka school can be divided into two branches: Svātantrika-Madhyamaka and Prāsaṅgika-Madhyamaka. The Yogācāra school can be divided into three: the phenomenological psychology of Vasubandhu and Asaṅga, the logical/epistemological branch of Dignāga and Dharmakīrti, and the metaphysical/ontological branch of Maitreya-Asaṅga, including the Yogācāra/*tathāgatagarbha* synthesis of Asaṅga's *Mahāyānasūtrālaṃkāra* and the purely *tathāgatagarbha* doctrine of Maitreya's *Uttaratantra*.[12] These Madhyamaka and Yogācāra schools share many doctrines in common, but differ in their interpretations of three major concepts: emptiness (*śūnyatā*), storehouse consciousness (*ālayavijñāna*), and Buddha nature (*tathāgathagarbha*). Their divergent interpretations of emptiness, in particular, have been topics of dispute in India, Tibet, and East Asia for centuries.

The Madhyamaka and Yogācāra systems rest on similar philosophical foundations. Proponents of both agree that composite phenomena are impermanent and arise in dependence on causes and conditions in accordance with the law of cause and effect. They accept a common Buddhist cosmology and agree that the impersonal functioning of dependent arising (*pratītyasamutpāda*) obviates the need for a creator god, cosmic consciousness, or a supreme being. Both agree that sentient beings possess the potential for awakening (*bodhi*) and accept the *Mahāparinirvāṇa Sūtra's* interpretation of this concept.[13] Both systems posit *śūnyatā* as the ultimate mode of existence of all phenomena and both advocate the middle way between the extremes of nihilism and eternalism. Both accept phenomena as existing conventionally and agree that phenomena do not exist as they appear to exist, that is, phenomena are devoid of independent, substantial existence and by nature are empty. Both schools consider that valid knowledge of phenomena and direct realization of emptiness are possible, and that direct insight into emptiness is a quality of all Buddhas and *bodhisattvas*. Although they may define *śūnyatā* differently, both schools concur with the *Vajraccedikāprajñāpāramitā Sūtra* when it says that the *bodhisattva*s are gifted with wisdom because, although they do not perceive things as truly existent, they still perceive things.[14] The commentary to this *sūtra* explains that *bodhisattvas* no longer assume the existence of a self (*ātman*), a continuity of existence (*sattva*), an enduring life force (*jīva*), or a person (*pudgala*).

Both the Madhyamaka and Yogācāra are systems of mental cultivation designed to counter the habitual tendency to concretize and essentialize experience, with the aim of achieving perfect awakening. In both systems, the knowledge and experience of ordinary beings is regarded as flawed because it is conditioned by the misconception that things exist as they appear, when in fact they do not. Ordinary perception is regarded as mistaken and misleading precisely because of sentient beings' habitual tendency to reify phenomena, especially their sense of self.

While the Madhyamaka and Yogācāra schools share much doctrinal common ground, they can also be distinguished at a number of points that are relevant to the topic of death and identity. First, these two schools emphasize different texts, on which they base their divergent interpretations. Followers of both systems regard the first "turning of the wheel" as a teaching intended for disciples of lesser capacity, known as *śrāvakas* (hearers), and regard the second and third turnings, based on the Prajñāpāramitā literature, as superior. The second turning of the wheel is regarded as definitive in Madhyamaka, however, whereas the third turning (*Laṅkāvatāra-sūtra* and related texts) is regarded as the final word in Yogācāra. Madhyamaka adherents reason that the Buddha taught the mind-only doctrine of the third turning as an expedient means (*upāya-kauśalya*), because explanations of the profound concept of *śūnyatā* were liable to a mistaken, nihilistic interpretation, whereas Yogācāra adherents regard the mind-only doctrine as superior.

A second point of difference is the Yogācāra theory of eight consciousnesses. In addition to the five sense consciousnesses and the mental consciousness (*mano-vijñāna*) accepted by other Buddhist schools, the Yogācāra system asserts two additional consciousnesses: *kliṣṭamanas* and *ālayavijñāna*. The seventh, *kliṣṭamanas*, is an afflicted type of consciousness that erroneously projects a sense of self. The eighth, *ālayavijñāna* (storehouse consciousness) is likened to a repository where the seeds or latent impressions of actions are stored until they mature. Even if the Yogācāra school does not represent an unqualified idealism (as Stefan Anacker and some others assert), the designations associated with the school—*cittamātra* (consciousness only or mind only), *vijñānavāda* (consciousness school), and *vijñāptimātra* (consciousness only)—indicate the central role consciousness plays in its exposition.

The chief doctrinal differences between Yogācāra and Madhyamaka concern the nature of ultimate reality—the concept of emptiness. In the Madhyamaka view, phenomena lack true existence, but
do exist conventionally. In the Yogācāra view, phenomena exist only
as they appear to consciousness, that is, they do not exist apart from
the consciousness that perceives them. From the Madhyamaka standpoint, to deny the existence of external objects is contradictory to
everyday experience—the conventional level of reality. From a Yogācāra
perspective, ultimately only consciousness exists. For adherents of this
view, to affirm the external existence of things would imply that there
was some substratum underlying phenomena, a view that would veer
toward the eternalist extreme.

Asaṅga argues at length for the mutual interdependence of names
and things, but he regards the ālayavijñāna as ultimately existent. He
regards the Madhyamaka position as nihilistic, claiming that if a thing
lacks ultimate existence, it cannot exist at all, since designations would
have no referent. In discussing the relationship of designations to their
objects, he holds that ultimate reality (pariṇipanna-svabhāva) is substan-
tially existent. He further asserts that the ultimate nature of things
(pāramārthika-svabhāva), although incomprehensible to ordinary beings,
can be cognized by beings who are free of discursive thought. Moreover, he objects to the theory of the two truths as a soteriological device.

Madhyamaka proponents define emptiness, the ultimate mode
of existence of phenomena, as the lack of inherent existence of all
phenomena, including emptiness itself. The lack of inherent existence
is explained as a non-affirming negation, one that posits nothing in its
place. Phenomena exist conventionally, as imputed by terms and concepts, but lack existence from their own side or "on their own accord,"
apart from causes and conditions. In the Madhyamaka view, there is
no substratum of reality or own-being of phenomena. Direct insight
into the emptiness of all phenomena, including emptiness, is a requi-
site for enlightenment.

Whereas in Madhyamaka proponents understand emptiness as
the lack of true existence of all phenomena, Yogācāra proponents define
emptiness as the absence of duality of subject and object. In his
Vimsatikā-vijñāptimātratā-siddhi, Vasubandhu equates emptiness with
selflessness (nairātmya), but defines emptiness specifically as the absence of any duality between the perceiving subject and the object that
is perceived. Seeing a distinction between subject and object, he asserts, is "a mistake of perception made by the ignorant." For Asaṅga,
the ultimate aim is a knowing that is free of such dualism: a "not-two"
realization. This ultimately leads to the subjective idealism that

Vasubandhu expresses in the *Vimsatikā*: "Everything is mind or representation only (*vijñapti-mātram-evaitat*), because there is the appearance of nonexistent objects, just as a person suffering from an ophthalmological disorder sees things which do not really exist."[15] In the *Laṅkāvatāra Sūtra* the Buddha is quoted as saying, "The external world is not, and the multiplicity of objects is what is seen of mind. Body, sense experience, dwelling place—I call just mind (*cittamātra*)."[16] A passage from the *Daśabhūmika Sūtra* also states: "These three realms [the realms of desire, corporeal matter, and immateriality] are nothing but mind."[17] On this view, the problem for sentient beings is that they mistakenly conceive objects to exist apart from consciousness. The fact that external objects appear to more than one person at the same time means that "we are all collectively hallucinating," as Liu Ming-Wood puts it. Madhyamaka followers reject this view, arguing that although our perceptions of external phenomena are distorted, external objects do exist, at least conventionally. In the Madhyamaka view, emptiness is not the absence of subject/object duality, but the lack of true existence of all phenomena.

Both the Madhyamaka and Yogācāra schools of Mahāyāna thought are predicated on earlier Buddhist ideas about death and identity. In both schools, the self and other composite phenomena are regarded as constantly changing constructs that appear in dependence upon a perceiving consciousness. In both schools, functional phenomena arise in dependence on causes and conditions and all eventually disintegrate. But there is disagreement between the Madhyamaka and Yogācāra schools about the nature of the perceiving consciousness and the status of what is perceived. In the nondual Yogācāra view, external objects do not exist even conventionally. In the Madhyamaka view, external objects exist conventionally, but ultimately they are empty of true existence. Yogācāra proponents claim that asserting the conventional reality of external objects leads to a substantialist view of the world and that denying the ultimate reality of consciousness leads to a nihilist view. Madhyamaka followers deny the Yogācāra claim that consciousness exists ultimately and that phenomena exist only as they appear to consciousness. These divergent views are significant for understanding the self that disintegrates at death.

Mind and Self: Collection and Continuity

The Mahāyāna perspective on the self is in agreement with early Buddhist theory: the five aggregates (*skandhas*) are the building blocks of the conventional person, but they are not ultimate, because these components themselves can be further deconstructed into smaller constituents. Early Mahāyāna proponents rejected the view that the *dharmas* (existent phenomena) are final realities or irreducible components of a person or thing, arguing instead that *dharmas* themselves are empty of true existence. Not only are the five aggregates absent of self, but so also are the constituents that make up the aggregates— body parts, molecules, atoms, electrons, and every iota of existence all the way down. This means that even the smallest component of the self lacks true existence. All the constituents are dependent phenomena like any other, arising in dependence on causes and conditions, and there is no soul, essence, or substratum that underlies any of it. Death is therefore simply a subsequent moment in a succession of momentary events that constitute the dependently arising person.

Yogācāra's chief concern is the nature of consciousness. Asaṅga elucidated three natures (*svabhāva*) or aspects of reality (*lakṣaṇāni*): (1) the conceptual, imagined, imputed, or illusory (*parikalpita*) aspect, which includes both imaginary phenomena and nonexistents; (2) the relative, dependent, or conventional (*paratantra*) aspect; and (3) the perfected or ultimate (*parinipanna*) aspect. The schema is intended to explain the process by which consciousness hypostatizes appearances and "creates the seeming reality of the subject/object duality."[18] As in other Buddhist schools, the root cause of cyclic existence (*saṃsāra*) is said to be a fundamental misconception about the nature of reality, or "the mode of existence of phenomena." The goal is to correct this misconception through critical analysis and meditation practice. In the Madhyamaka school, the fundamental misconception of reality is the illusion of true existence, whereas in the Yogācāra school the fundamental misconception is the illusion of duality between the perceiver and the perceived. In both schools, awakening means gaining direct insight into the true nature of reality.[19]

In the *Treatise on the Three Aspects*, Vasubandhu says,

> The relative aspect of experience is simply experience as it appears; the imagined aspect of experience is that same experience (which is all there is) appearing in the mode of a subject—a person—cognizing objects. Both of these are called "imagination of the unreal" because, ontologically speaking, there are neither persons nor objects; there is only experience.[20]

Paul J. Griffiths clarifies that the relative and imagined aspects of experience are not ontologically distinct; the latter is simply the perception of the former through the dualistic lens of the subject-object dichotomy. Nor is the perfected aspect of experience ontologically distinct, since "the relative is all there is." The perfected aspect is simply the enlightened experience of Buddhas, free of subject-object dualism.[21]

In Buddhist systems other than Yogācāra, consciousness or awareness always has an object: to be aware is to be conscious of *something*. This view is most explicitly formulated by the Vaibhāṣika school. Each moment of consciousness is said to have its specific object and no moment of consciousness lacks an object. In the Yogācāra system, however, the *ālayavijñāna* (storehouse consciousness) is said to exist inherently even in the absence of an object. Phenomena other than the *ālayavijñāna* are regarded as mental events (*citta*) or representations (*vijñāpti*) that exist without corresponding external objects. This consciousness-centered ontology therefore came to be known as the "mind only" (*cittamātra*) or "mere consciousness" (*vijñāptivāda*) view. Scholarly opinion is divided on whether Yogācāra is a strictly idealist position and the debate centers on whether only consciousness exists, or whether consciousness is all we can access.[22]

In the Yogācāra school, the theory of *ālayavijñāna* helps explain the workings of *karma* in the absence of an enduring self. Actions of body, speech, and mind are said to leave subtle imprints (*vāsanā*) or "seeds" (*bīja*) on the *ālayavijñāna* that may ripen in subsequent moments of consciousness. The *ālayavijñāna* is a continuing underlying consciousness that serves as a storehouse for the imprints or impressions of physical, verbal, and mental actions. These imprints, likened to "scents," are akin to habitual tendencies, predispositions, or propensities for creating similar actions in future lifetimes. Paul J. Griffiths views this theory as a philosophical construct to help reconcile "the experienced facts of the continuity of personal identity, such things as memory, continuity of character traits, the continuing sense that each person thinks of himself as identifiably an individual, identifiably different from other individuals and identifiably the same person as he was in the past," with a metaphysics that denies the existence of enduring individuals and events.[23]

In addition to providing a locus for karmic seeds, the *ālayavijñāna* is also a way of explaining the continuity of individuated identity from one lifetime to the next. According to the Yogācāra line of reasoning, the consciousness that leaves the body at death must be the *ālayavijñāna*, because the *ālayavijñāna* is the only type of consciousness that can operate without objects. Other Buddhist schools reject the *ālayavijñāna* and the notion of a consciousness that exists without objects. For them, the mental consciousness (*manovijñāna*) is perfectly capable of continuing after death and there is no need to posit an additional consciousness. The same reasoning that is used to refute the existence of a self-reflective consciousness (*svasaṃvedanā*, self-knower) is used to refute the idea of *ālayavijñāna*. Consciousness is simply conscious; there is no need to posit an additional, self-aware consciousness. Similarly there is no need to posit an *ālayavijñāna* to explain the relationships between the six consciousnesses; the six consciousnesses are simply conscious or aware. The idea of a foundational consciousness is rejected on the same grounds as the notion of a substratum underlying phenomenal existence.

In the *Yogācārabhūmi*, Asaṅga outlines eight negative consequences of not positing the *ālayavijñāna*. Without the *ālayavijñāna*, he says, (1) it is impossible to appropriate a new body; (2) the sense consciousnesses can neither originate nor function; (3) clear mental consciousness is impossible; (4) it is impossible to explain the successive occurrence of incompatible events (e.g., virtuous and nonvirtuous thoughts in the mental continuum); (5) mental experience is impossible; (6) physical experience is impossible; (7) cessation (e.g., for a living *ārhat*) is impossible; and (8) death is impossible. The *Abhidharmasauccayabhāsya* (available in both Tibetan and Chinese translations) explains that the *ālayavijñāna* is necessary because it serves as the "appropriator" of a body in the next life.

For opponents of the Yogācāra position, the *ālayavijñāna* is simply the self in disguise. Even though the *ālayavijñāna* is described merely as a repository of karmic imprints and is subject to the law of cause and effect, because it endures beyond death, it resembles a permanent entity and is therefore at variance with early Buddhist theories of no-self and impermanence. Moreover, as Griffiths points out, the *ālayavijñāna* does not satisfy "standard Buddhist definitions of consciousness as something which cognizes, something which has an intentional object,"[24] instead consisting merely of extremely subtle "seeds" of awareness that are destined to "ripen" at some subsequent time, in conjunction with causes and conditions. Neither conscious nor material, the nature and status of the *ālayavijñāna* is ambiguous and far too closely approximates a self to be acceptable to the adherents of other Buddhist schools.

In the Madhyamaka school, the self exists conventionally but lacks ultimate reality. Because the conventional self and its component parts all arise in dependence on causes and conditions, they are said to be empty of true existence. Cause and effect still function for the conventional self, but there is nothing substantial to serve as a basis for clinging, attachment, and the other mental afflictions. The conventional self and its ultimate nature (emptiness) function in necessary and contingent relationship to one another, mirroring the contingent relationship between dependent arising (*pratītyasamutpāda*) and emptiness (*śūnyatā*). According to this school, the theory of karma elucidated above functions just as well without an *ālayavijñāna*. Actions of body, speech, and mind leave their imprints on successive moments of consciousness and the mental continuum—comprised of these moments—continues to a subsequent rebirth, but without an *ālayavijñāna*. Not only is there no basis for positing an *ālayavijñāna*, but such a concept could too easily be misconstrued as an enduring self.

Tathāgathagarbha: Self in a New Guise?

In addition to the *ālayavijñāna*, the Yogācāra schools emphasize the concept of *tathāgathagarbha*, the "embryo of the Tathāgata" or Buddha nature. There are several distinguishable phases of Yogācāra thought in India: the early works of Vasubhandu and Asaṅga, the later works of Dignāga and Dharmakīrti, and the texts attributed to Maitreya-Asaṅga. It is especially the latter works that emphasize the *tathāgathagarbha* concept, most notably the *Uttaratantra*. The earliest description of the *tathāgathagarbha* is found in the *Ratnagotravibhāga*, which dates from around the third century. The *tathāgathagarbha* doctrine came into full flower in China and was a key element in the formulation of Tiantai, Huayan, and Chan thought. Implicit in this concept is the belief that each and every sentient being not only can, but eventually will become a fully awakened Buddha.

The nature of the *tathāgathagarbha* is variously interpreted either as the potential for enlightenment within sentient beings, or the enlightened mind that is inherent within beings and just temporarily obscured. The tension between these two views is already apparent in the *Tathāgathagarbha-sūtra* itself. Proponents of both views agree that sentient beings possess the seed or "embryo" of enlightenment (*tathāgathagarbha*) that will manifest when the delusions that obscure it are removed. Whether the *tathāgathagarbha* is merely a potentiality or is enlightenment itself, in either case, the *tathāgathagarbha* can easily be misconstrued as being ultimately existent—a sort of surrogate for the self—as is boldly asserted in the Mahāyāna *Parinirvāṇa Sūtra*. Some argue that this statement, attributed to the Buddha in the *sūtra*, is not meant to be taken literally. According to this view, the *tathāgathagarbha* is merely a skillful means (*upāya*) to expedite awakening among those who either cling to the belief in a self or veer toward a nihilist view of the self.

Although the *ālayavijñāna* discussed by Asaṅga and Vasubandhu seems primarily a convenient way of explaining how the imprints of actions are transmitted from one lifetime to the next, the *Laṅkāvatāra-sūtra* appears to equate *tathāgathagarbha* with *ālayavijñāna*. The assertion that the *tathāgathagarbha* is inherently existent invited the criticism of Madhyamaka proponents, for whom any assertion of inherent existence is comparable to an assertion of an ongoing permanent self (*ātman*) underlying the *skandhas*. Together, these two concepts—an inherently existent *tathāgathagarbha* and a storehouse consciousness (Tib: *kun gshi rnam she*, mind basis of all)—clearly left the door open for the reintroduction of a substantive notion of self.

Chandrakīrti, the renowned seventh-century interpreter of Nāgārjuna, disputes the Yogācāra view that only consciousness exists ultimately and that external phenomena exist only as they appear to consciousness. He rejects the *ālayavijñāna* and the notion of any ultimately existent consciousness, and makes the point that appearances could not arise without the existence of external phenomena as their causes. For Chandrakīrti, each moment of consciousnesses is a momentary event that arises in dependence on a previous moment of consciousnesses. On his view, if the *ālayavijñāna* is not capable of cognizing an object, then it is not, properly speaking, a consciousness, because a consciousness by definition arises when a physical or mental sense base encounters its appropriate object. If there are no external objects, if only mental phenomena exist, and physical phenomena are merely appearances, sentient beings would not feel physical pain, but they do. The *ālayavijñāna* is rejected because it is superfluous, and subjective idealism is rejected because it is contradicted by empirical experience. Consciousness is simply conscious and does not require any substratum for its functioning.

Indian Buddhist texts describe a functional dependency between the person and the aggregates. The person is seen as a conceptual construct that arises on the basis of a perceived continuity of the aggregates. When the aggregates disintegrate at death, consciousness also begins a process of disintegration or transformation that entails a disintegration of the illusion of self. In both Yogācāra and Madhyamaka, the self is merely a mental construct, a convenient fiction that is functional on the conventional level. Death nevertheless has a powerful impact, because the ordinary person strongly identifies with the illusion of self, grasps at the self as being real, and fears its disintegration. The stronger a person's habitual tendency to identify with the self, the more suffering the person experiences at the time of death, as the aggregates disintegrate and the illusion of self shatters.

When the concept of *ālayavijñāna* is introduced, exegetists are careful to reiterate that the self has no independent reality, but is merely an illusion projected upon the aggregates. They explain that the imprints of actions, including imprints of the habitual tendency to grasp at the self, are simply stored in the *ālayavijñāna*. If the *ālayavijñāna* is transitory, it can be regarded as merely another name for the mental consciousness in its capacity to store these imprints, in the same way that the mental consciousness is understood to function in other Buddhist schools. If the *ālayavijñāna* is conceived to be a substratum of consciousness, then it takes on a more substantial quality and can easily be mistaken for a self.

In both Yogācāra and Madhyamaka systems, the world of things is mentally constructed, but there is a fundamental difference of opinion between the two schools concerning the existence of external objects and the ontological status of mind. The Yogācāra contends that phenomena are entirely dependent upon the perceiving consciousness; objects exist *only* as they appear to the mind. The Madhyamaka agrees that the appearance of phenomena are dependent on consciousness, since phenomena are literally "objects of consciousness," but cannot be said to be mere appearances because they do exist conventionally. Both schools accept the theory of karma and agree that the "imprints" of actions ripen in this and future lifetimes, but the Yogācāra contends that these imprints are stored in the *ālayavijñāna*, whereas the Madhyamaka refutes the concept of the *ālayavijñāna* as unnecessary and liable to misinterpretation as an inherently existent consciousness that continues from one rebirth to the next.

The tendency for unenlightened individuals to grasp at the illusion of a self is natural, since individuals habitually identify with their bodies and minds. The notion of *ālayavijñāna*, especially in conjunction with the theory of *tathāgatagarbha*, satisfies the perceived need for stability and self-identity and is easier to accept than a notion of self as merely contingent. Even when the idea of a solid self is denied intellectually, there may still be a strong instinctual tendency to conceive of the self as something enduring. Once the mental continuum becomes substantiated in the form of the *ālayavijñāna* substrate, however, it is not much of a leap to a more inclusive subjective ontology, such as a cosmic consciousness or subjective monism. For this reason, an understanding of the nature of consciousness and individual continuity is critical for understanding the nature of death and moral agency, and for applying this understanding to a critical analysis of bioethical issues from a Buddhist perspective.

Chapter 6

Death and Enlightenment in Tibet

The Tibetan Plateau is situated directly north of India and Nepal, separated by the enormity of the Himalayan mountain range that stretches from east to west. In this sparsely populated high-altitude region, the indigenous religious beliefs and practices known as Bön centered around the propitiation of deities in the natural environment. Due to the snowy Himalayan peaks and distance, it was not until the seventh century CE that Buddhist culture began to make a major impact in Tibet. Several miraculous portents are said to have drawn certain Tibetans' attention to Buddhism as early as the first century CE, but it was not until the reign of Songtsen Gampo (618–650)—through marriage alliances with princesses from Nepal and China—that sacred images and monasteries began to proliferate in Tibet. King Songtsen Gampo sent the scholar Tönmi Sambhota to India to devise a script for the Tibetan language in order to facilitate the translation of Sanskrit Buddhist texts. Subsequent kings continued to send Tibet's brightest young scholars to India to study, to invite teachers, and to acquire Buddhist texts and commentaries. Thus began a centuries-long process of translating the Buddhist canon into Tibetan.

The Buddhism that prevailed in India during the period when Buddhist literature was transmitted to Tibet (between the eighth and tenth centuries) included two major discernible streams: the analytical systems of philosophical tenets that flourished in the great monastic universities, and the esoteric tantric meditation systems that were practiced in great secrecy in mountain caves and other solitary spots. Under royal patronage, the Tibetans exerted enormous energy to import

Buddhist texts and teachings of various traditions and lineages, and then spent the next thousand years analyzing and practicing them.

Bön and Tibetan Buddhism

The religious traditions of pre-Buddhist Tibet are collectively known today as Bön. These indigenous traditions have absorbed so many Buddhist ideas and practices over the course of time that they have in many respects become nearly indistinguishable from Buddhism. These confluences, combined with the lack of early historical documentation, make it extremely difficult to get an accurate idea of Bön civilization as it existed prior to the advent of Buddhism. We do know that pre-Buddhist shamanistic traditions were deeply concerned with the spirits of the dead. Skilled ritual specialists carried out elaborate funerary rites and were believed capable of discerning traces of the dead in substances, after a person's consciousness had departed. Bön priests formulated three hundred sixty ways of dying, four ways of preparing graves, and eighty-one ways of taming evil spirits.[1] Offerings to the dead, the sacrifice of particular animals, and other rituals were performed to ensure a blissful afterlife for the souls of the dead. It was also believed that souls could be exorcised by funerary specialists to benefit the dead. These early beliefs and practices reveal an early interest in the liminal aspects of death and could explain the Tibetan Buddhist emphasis on death and dying in subsequent centuries. Even today, Bön practitioners in some Tibetan cultural areas continue to perform these funeral rites.[2]

Sky burial, a Tibetan practice still in evidence in Tibet today, most likely springs from the Bön tradition. In sky burial, on a particular day that is determined by divination, the corpse of the deceased is chopped into pieces and fed to the birds. This unique practice, which may appear disrespectful of the dead, is performed as a final act of generosity. Since rotting flesh is of no use to the deceased and the consciousness of the deceased is believed to have already left the body, it is considered an act of merit to donate the flesh to animals, especially "higher" animals, such as birds. Disposing of the dead in this manner surely reflects the environment, because in the mountainous terrain of Tibet, the earth was too hard to dig graves and fuel for cremation was scarce and costly. Cremation was only an option for wealthy or illustrious people such as renowned lamas. Rituals carried out to determine the karmic destiny of a dead person or to exorcise troublesome spirits apparently trace their roots to Bön and similar shamanic practices, and are performed even today.

Shamanic practices never died out in Tibetan societies and many of their complex rituals for death and other aspects of life persisted long after Buddhism was introduced. Geoffrey Samuel suggests that, prior to Buddhism, funerary rituals were focused on protecting the surviving community from the spirits of the dead,[3] whereas after Buddhism was introduced emphasis shifted to the welfare of the dead person in the afterlife. Although Buddhism is well-known for rejecting the notion of an enduring soul, Samten Karmay argues that "Buddhism was never able to suppress the concept of soul in Tibet."[4] The concept of *la* may be translated as soul, spirit, life force, or life essence. A person's *la* (*bla*) is not the same as the self, but is specifically associated with an individual. In Tibetan culture, it is believed that a person's *la* can wander away and be lost, leading to psychological disorientation or psychosis. In such an eventuality, a qualified religious specialist (shaman) may be requested to perform specific rituals to lure the *la* back into the person's body. A talisman, often a piece of turquoise, is then worn to ensure that the *la* does not wander off again.

La is a concept not only associated with human beings, such as a personal life force, but also with animals, natural elements, and places. At the time of birth, the *la* appears in conjunction with five other deities, representing life, female, male, enemy, and locality. Just as Hawaiians plant a breadfruit tree at the birth of a child, in some regions Tibetans plant a tree, usually a juniper, which they call a "*la* tree" (*la shing*).[5] The *la* is related to fortune in this life rather than to liberation, and does not seem to be related to rebirth.[6] Geoffrey Samuel says that, "The *la* can leave the body, weakening one's life and exposing one to harm. It can also be affected by damaging or destroying its external resting-place."[7] The *la* must be protected from harmful influences and "returned" through rituals if stolen. The fact that rituals such as these continue up to the present day in Tibetan societies is evidence that a covert theory of soul (*la*) has endured since pre-Buddhist times and continues to coexist with the Buddhist concept of no-self.

With regard to death, there is considerable common ground between Bön and Tibetan Buddhism. Both draw analogies between death and sleep, death and dreaming, and exhort practitioners to maintain total awareness as the internal and external signs of death are encountered. Both Bön and Tibetan Buddhism speak of: (1) *phowa* (*'pho ba*) practice (transference of consciousness), (2) visions in the *bardo* (intermediate state), (3) prayers for the dead for forty-nine days, and (4) liberation in the *bardo*. But there are also some conceptual differences between Bön and Tibetan Buddhism. For example, Bön speaks of the Six Clear Knowledges of: (1) death, (2) cause and effect, (3) complete knowledge, (4) clear light of the *bardo*, (5) nature of the mind, and (6) *trikāya* (similar to the Buddhist *trikāya*, "three bodies of the Buddha"). It also mentions the Six Recollections on: (1) past lives, (2) stages of the *bardo*, (3) consciousness as without support, (4) the master's instructions, (5) visions as mental projections, and (6) the pure essence of mind that opens onto one's *yidam* (meditational deity).[8] Instead of four or six *bardos* as in Tibetan Buddhism, however, Bön speaks of just three, each of which corresponds to a different level of practitioner: superior, average, and inferior. The superior practitioner is one who dies with total awareness of the absolute view [emptiness], liberating the mind into the essential nature of reality like "a snowflake dissolving in the ocean." The uniquely Tibetan Buddhist meditation practice called *chö* (*chod*), "cutting through" may have been influenced by Bön. In the visualization practice of *chö*, one perfects the virtue of generosity by donating one's own severed limbs and internal organs to hungry ghosts and spirits, accompanied by the rhythm of drums and lyrical chanting. *Chö* practice presages the physical dissolution that awaits all sentient beings at death and helps nurture both detachment and compassion for the needy.

The Ephemeral Nature of Life

Newcomers are often struck by the centrality of death in the Tibetan Buddhist tradition. Images of Yama, the Lord of Death, greet visitors at the door of most Tibetan temples. Beginning meditators are taught to meditate on the impermanence of life and to reflect that from the moment of birth, death stalks "like a murderer with poised sword." To visualize one's own rotting corpse and the dissolution of body and mind at the time of death engenders insight into the impermanence of life. This insight then acts as an antidote to laziness and attachment. One learns to direct the eighty-four thousand winds of the body into the central psychic channel, through the crown of the head, and toward a rebirth in a Pure Land. Another method of teaching impermanence is the ritual of creating a three-dimensional sand *maṇḍala* symbolizing the "pure land" of the enlightened being that all sentient beings are capable of becoming. After being carefully constructed, the *maṇḍala* is destroyed and thrown into moving water to symbolize the ephemeral quality of all life. Ritual instruments used in the *cham* (meditative motion, also referred to as monastic dance) and other tantric rituals symbolize cutting through the attachment to self. In various ways, each of these practices offers methods to demolish misconceptions about the self. Symbolically, ego identification is transcended on three levels: (1) the outer, symbolizing external form, (2) the inner, symbolizing the emotions, and (3) the secret, symbolizing the subtle mind and body.

Other examples of practices related to death are the visualization techniques described in the tantric texts that were transmitted from India. These visualization techniques are still a mainstay of Tibetan Buddhist practice today. In meditative experience, one imagines oneself to be an awakened being, free of all unwholesome mind states and endowed with all enlightened qualities, a practice that is believed to naturally purify the mind of all defilements. The aim of the developing stage of tantric practice is to purify birth, death, and the intermediate state between death and rebirth.[9] The conscious and continuous visualization of oneself as an awakened being is thought to eliminate unproductive and unwholesome states of consciousness, or "impure manifestations," during the critical intermediate stage. The process of visualizing oneself as an enlightened being intimately illustrates the mutable nature of self-identity and the potential of the mind to create alternative realities. By identifying with enlightened figures in many forms, female and male, one gains an understanding that gender and other aspects of personal identity are constructs and not fixed. In this way, one gains insight into the reconfiguration that occurs at death and prepares to allow only that which is truly authentic to remain.

A huge corpus of literature generally referred to under the rubric of *Lamrim* (*The Graduated Path to Enlightenment*) arose in Tibet to facilitate study and meditation on key Buddhist concepts; meditation on death and dying is among the principal topics. The texts provide instructions for actual meditation practice, including contemplation on the inevitability of death and the stages of the dying process. In the texts are many slogans designed to remind the practitioner throughout the meditation that death is definite, yet the time of death is indefinite, and at the time of death only Dharma practice will be of benefit. These meditations on death and dying are done repeatedly to help practitioners develop detachment and equanimity, and to prepare them to meet death calmly and constructively.

Death forces us to confront the self's mortality, what B. Alan Wallace calls "life's oldest illusion," and recognize how we are "enmeshed in the chain of trivial concerns that fill daily life."[10] Attitudes toward death are thus closely connected to a sense of personal identity, because death represents the loss of a person's familiar identifications, especially identification with this body and mind. Strong emotions such as anger or attachment to friends and possessions are viewed as serious impediments to mindful, meaningful dying and causes for disagreeable future rebirths.

From a Tibetan perspective, it is assumed that the series of mental events or moments of mental consciousness that comprise an individual's mental continuum continues on after the physical elements disintegrate and eventually is linked to a new locus of physical components. This cycle repeats endlessly—each successive rebirth bringing a different identity, with unique propensities as a result of its karmic ledger. The nature of consciousness is therefore central to the Tibetan Buddhist understanding of death and its consequences.

In the Tibetan Buddhist worldview, the "person" is a concatenation of physical and mental components or momentary events. All functional phenomena belong to one of three mutually distinct yet interrelated categories: matter (*kanthā*), consciousnesses (*jñāna*), and nonassociated compositional factors (*viprayukta-saṃskāra*).[11] Actions of body, speech, and mind create imprints on successive moments of consciousness, and lie dormant in the mental continuum until conditions are conducive to their ripening, creating the conditions for further actions of body, speech, and mind. Each moment of consciousness conditions successive moments of consciousness. Actions of body, speech, and mind thus generate further actions, whether wholesome or unwholesome. Consciousness does not simply cease at the time of death, but gives rise to subsequent moments of consciousness. These causally connected moments of consciusness are believed to continue into an intermediate state (*bardo*) between the moment of death and the moment of one's next rebirth. Because the moment of consciousness at the time of death acts as the cause of subsequent moments of consciousness in the next state of existence, the quality of one's consciousness at the time of death is critical. The quality of one's final moment in one lifetime—peaceful, angry, loving, spiteful—influences the quality of the first moment of one's next existence. Consequently, Tibetan practitioners train their minds to remain calm and attentive during the stages of the dying process and the intermediate state, in the belief that this will lead to a more fortunate rebirth.

Rehearsing One's Dying

In the harsh climate of Tibet, death is a constant threat. Temperatures dip far below freezing and life is generally at the mercy of the elements. Tibetan practitioners take the Buddha's teachings on death very seriously. At the portal to the next life awaits Yama, the Lord of Death. Eager to snap up the unsuspecting, he metaphorically weighs the

deceased's former actions, punishing evil deeds with terrifying consequences and rewarding good deeds with a happy destiny in the next
life. The physical components of the person disintegrate within a given
time span, determined by the quality of one's spiritual practice and
the level of realization attained. The consciousness of an experienced
practitioner may remain in meditation for some time and delay the
decomposition of the body. After the physical components disintegrate, what becomes of them is inconsequential, thus to offer the flesh
and ground bones to vultures is not grotesque, but rather a commend-
able act of generosity. *Chö*, the ritual practice of offering one's body
parts to spirits in meditation, appears to be a rehearsal for the dis-
memberment that follows actual death. To witness a sky burial is a
singular reminder of human mortality and the dispersion of corporeal
elements that awaits all living creatures.

Tibetan texts give accounts of *yogis* who pass away leaving
only their hair and fingernails behind, and ascend to a Pure Land in
a rainbow body. These highly accomplished *yogis* are presumed to
be *bodhisattvas*, selfless beings who work for three countless aeons to
accumulate the merit and wisdom needed for perfect awakening.
These *yogis* instantiate the enlightened quest of the Buddha by meditating and dying in lotus posture, far away from human society.
They do not fulfill the twelve deeds that characterize the life of a
fully enlightened Buddha, but they are thought to achieve final enlightenment in one of the many Pure Lands after death. By demonstrating tangible spiritual achievements and thereby the effectiveness
of Buddhist practice, these *yogis* become archetypes with enormous
social and religious significance.

All Buddhist schools assert that the mental continuum, being
nonmaterial, may travel from one life to the next without any time
lapse, especially in the case of a sudden accident. In contrast to
Buddhaghoṣa, who argues that rebirth *necessarily* takes place immediately, Tibetans believe that the consciousness transverses an intermediate state (*bardo*) for a period of up to forty-nine days. The *bardo* being
seeks an appropriate rebirth in a series of seven intervals, each up to
seven days in length. At each stage, the *bardo* being assumes an identity that presages the form it will take in the next state of existence. At
the end of each interval, if an appropriate body is not found, the being
experiences a "small death" and takes birth in another intermediate
state (*bardo*). Each *bardo* being is said to take a form similar to the
identity it will assume in the next rebirth. These changing identities
can be seen as analogs of the series of identities an individual assumes
over the course of innumerable lifetimes, from beginningless time up

to final enlightenment. Under the influence of defilements, particularly sexual desire, the mental consciousness of an ordinary being eventually is attracted to a couple in sexual union. As a result of this attraction, the consciousness enters the mother's womb and conception occurs.

The term *bardo* (Skt: *antarābhāva*) is most commonly used to refer to the intermediate state between death in one lifetime and rebirth in the next. In fact, the term may denote one of six intermediate states (*bardo*): (1) birth (*skye ba'i bar do*), (2) dream (*rmi lam gyi bar do*), (3) meditative concentration (*bsam gten gyi bar do*), (4) death (*'chi ka'i bar do*), (5) the afterdeath state of reality itself (*chos nyi bar do*, Skt: *dharmatā*), and (6) rebirth or "becoming" (*srid pa'i bar do*). The *bardo* of birth includes all the experiences and actions of waking reality, from birth until death. The *bardo* of dream includes all experiences and mental events during sleep. The *bardo* of meditative concentration includes all mental events and realizations experienced during meditation practice. The *bardo* of death includes all events during the process of dying and the moment of death. The afterdeath *bardo* of reality itself includes all the mental events experienced once one regains consciousness after death. And the *bardo* of rebirth includes all the experiences involved in seeking an appropriate next birth.[12] The *bardo* of rebirth ceases with the *bardo* of birth, and the cycle begins again.

Navigating the Journey to the Next Life

As death approaches, the dying person is encouraged to reflect on the impermanent, suffering, self-less nature of the mind and all other composite phenomena, as described in the early Buddhist texts. In the Tibetan tradition, a person who is sufficiently trained will meditate on the luminous, empty, knowing nature of the mind, and be prepared to recognize the clear light nature of the mind when it appears at the final moment of the dying process. A practitioner receives instructions on the stages of the dying process and how to recognize the physiological, psychological, and visionary indicators that occur at each stage. If the practitioner has rehearsed these practices and become thoroughly familiar with the stages of dying, it is possible not only to avoid unfortunate "migrations" after death, but also to achieve high spiritual realizations, including enlightenment, during the stages of the dying process and the intermediate state.

Tibetan medical lore explains how to determine the time of death by analyzing the urine of the critically ill patient and by reading the death pulse.[13] Of the four medical *tantras*, the second describes the signs of death in detail.[14] A composite of gross and subtle winds (*bar do rlung lus*, Skt: *antarābhavayukāya*) is said to continue during the intermediate state after death. Death is regarded as a process, rather than a unitary event. The subtle winds and subtle mind that continue after physical death are the basis for the only semblance of identity that survives an individual's death.

In his translation of Padmasambhava's *Book of Natural Liberation Through Understanding in the Between* [*Liberation through Hearing in the Bardo*], Robert A. F. Thurman says:

> Western science holds that a "flatline" on the EEG means cessation of heartbeat and brain activity, and therefore represents death. The illusion of the subjective "I" in the individual consciousness, assumed by materialists to correspond with the presence of brain wave activity, should cease with the cessation of brain waves. Yet the picture of death as nothing in consciousness is not a scientific finding. It is a conceptual notion. There are many cases of people being revived after "flatlining" for some time, and they report intense subjective experiences.[15]

Some people do survive flatlining and may report their experiences.[16] Thurman applies Blaise Pascal's wager: If there is nothing after death, well and good; if there is something, we will not regret being prepared for it. Thurman describes *karma* as a process of psychobiological evolution and Buddhist practice as the evolutionary technology needed to die lucidly and then to skillfully traverse the intermediate state.

Tibetan Funerary Practices

Among Buddhists, purifying the mind, absolving negative karma, creating positive karma, and loosening the bonds that bind an individual to the world are concerns not only for the living, but also for those in the intermediate state after death. *Liberation through Hearing in the Bardo* (*Bar do thos grol*), the well-known instruction manual for guiding the dying through the *bardo* between death and rebirth, is often an integral part of funeral rituals. The text, attributed to Padmasambhava and discovered by Karma Lingpa (1326–1386), is an example of the hidden treasure text (*gter ma*) genre of literature associated with the Nyingma tradition. The text guides the dying in: (1) recognizing the fundamental clear light nature of the mind at the time of death; (2) recognizing the true nature of the wrathful and peaceful images that appear to the mind; and (3) achieving liberation from rebirth. Just as a prisoner on death row may experience a spiritual breakthrough, the intensity of the experience of dying can serve as a catalyst for spiritual awakening. It is believed that a highly competent practitioner may even achieve enlightenment in the *bardo*.

The Tibetan Buddhist tradition teaches that no matter how defiled one's ordinary consciousness may be, at its center lies a core of luminosity—the potential to become a fully enlightened Buddha. To realize the luminous nature of the mind at the moment of death is itself a liberation from the delusions that obscure the true nature of the mind. The luminous, ultimately nonconceptual nature of the mind is also alluded to in early texts such as the *Anguttara Nikāya*. Although this understanding may also be developed through meditation practice while one is alive, the dying process presents an ideal opportunity to discover the clear light nature of the mind—the primary identifying aspect of all sentient beings. Without proper preparation, an individual is propelled after death into a new rebirth totally as a result of *karma* and afflictive emotions. Therefore, practitioners make efforts to gain control of the mind and train in navigating the stages of dying beforehand, so as to remain calm and aware during the "journey" and achieve a desirable rebirth.

Actual practices vary according to the individual and the lineage. If a person has been a practitioner of a particular meditational deity (*yi dam*) or lineage of transmission, it is common to incorporate that practice and lineage into funeral proceedings. The goal is to achieve enlightenment "in this life, in this very body," but in case one is not able to accomplish this goal, there still remains the opportunity to direct one's consciousness to a Pure Land after death. An extremely proficient adept can effect rebirth in a Pure Land even without experiencing the *bardo*. Such adepts are said to be "deathless"; the coarse physical body transforms into a pure rainbow body and leaves no corpse behind. When this occurs, rainbows appear in the clear blue sky and the practitioner's hair and fingernails are all that is left behind in the meditation cell. Reports of such phenomena are common in Tibetan cultural lore.

Phowa: Transference of Consciousness

The uniquely Tibetan meditation practice known as *phowa*, "transference of consciousness," is a means of preparing for the journey to the next rebirth. By learning to control the winds of the body and how to consciously direct them through the psychic channels, practitioners learn to successfully guide their consciousness from this life to a rebirth in a Pure Land at the moment of death. For one sufficiently trained in *phowa*, death is the culmination of the practice. Not only can one avoid an unfortunate future rebirth, but a competent *phowa* practitioner is able to collect the eighty-four thousand winds of the body into the central psychic channel and direct the subtle mind to a rebirth in a "fortunate migration" or a Pure Land.

The *Yoga of Consciousness Transference* text by Tsechokling Yeshe Gyaltsen, the *guru* of the eighth Dalai Lama, describes a *phowa* practice that focuses on Maitreya Buddha "wherein all energies of the body are withdrawn just as at the time of death and a meditational experience equivalent to death is aroused."[17] The preliminaries to *phowa* practice include the elimination of nonvirtuous mental states and the cultivation of virtuous ones through: (1) generating *bodhicitta,* the enlightened attitude of wishing to achieve the state of perfect Buddhahood in order to liberate all sentient beings from suffering; (2) accumulating merit; (3) meditating repeatedly on *bodhicitta;* (4) eliminating negativity through purification practices; and (5) aspiring never to become separated from the *bodhicitta.*[18] In the actual practice session, one first visualizes Maitreya Buddha in Tuṣita Pure Land, surrounded by countless *bodhisattvas,* and then invokes him to manifest at the place of practice. Next one recites liturgies of offering, purification, invocation, and dedication, and visualizes a nectar of purification and blessings streaming from Maitreya into oneself. One visualizes blocking the subsidiary pathways of the body and invites Maitreya to the crown of one's head. Concentrating on a drop of light in the central energy channel as being in the nature of one's own mind, one invokes Maitreya, who fills the central channel with brilliant light. One then repeatedly visualizes the light drop at one's heart, along with the vital energies, shooting up until it reaches the crown aperture and then descending. In order to achieve the signs of perfect accomplishment, the practitioner must bear in mind the illusory nature of the self, the consciousness, and the process of transference, also known as the emptiness of "the three circles."[19]

As the actual time of death approaches, one accumulates merit by giving away all one's possessions and then, lying on the right side in the "lion posture," begins the practice. Great care must be taken in the practice of *phowa*, however, to ensure that one's consciousness does not accidently leave the body before one's life span is exhausted. Because the practitioner is consciously identifying with the meditational deity, to eject the consciousness from the body and die prematurely is not only equivalent to suicide—a serious ethical transgression—but also slays the deity that is the object of identification. It is a widely shared value that Dharma practitioners should attempt to prolong their lives in order to fulfill their spiritual objectives. Long life initiations or empowerments (*tse dbang*) are among the numerous ritual enactments to prevent untimely death and prolong life. Collectively, these practices are designed to "cheat death."[20]

Chö: Deconstructing the Illusory Self

The Mahāyāna teachings emphasize compassion, *bodhicitta*, and meditation techniques that erode the self-cherishing attitude. One well-known practice for eradicating self-cherishing and perfecting the virtue of generosity is *chö*, or "cutting through." In this practice, one visualizes cutting off one's limbs and other body parts, and symbolically offering them to hungry ghosts and other beings in need:

> The *Chöd* rites were reputed to have been begun in the eleventh century by the Tibetan female mystic, Machig Labdron. In the myth surrounding her life, a male yogi in India transferred his consciousness into the body of a female foetus in Tibet and she was born with miraculous powers. It was during her reading of the *Prajñāpāramitā* that she achieved insight pertaining to the emptiness of all things, and developed the practice which uses visualizations of demons to overcome fears and dispel the notion of a belief in a "self." In the practice, the meditator beats the rhythm of the chant with a large hand-held drum and simultaneously rings a bell, which is said to represent the feminine. At intervals a thigh bone trumpet is blown to summon the demons to a feast of the meditator's ego.[21]

The practice aims at cutting through the delusions of the mind, particularly attachment to the body and the illusion of an independent self.

The practice of *chö* that developed in Tibet has its roots in early Buddhist texts, specifically the Jātaka tales, the past life legends about Buddha Śākyamuni. In a past life as a *bodhisattva*, the Buddha is believed to have cut off the flesh from his own thigh and given it to a hungry tigress to save her and her cubs from starvation. Namo Buddha, the sacred site in Nepal that commemorates this compassionate deed, is a popular destination for Buddhist pilgrims from around the world even today.

In one of the few academic studies of *chö*, Janet Gyatso traces the practice to four main Indian sources: Āryadeva's *Tsigs bcad*, Nāro's *Ro sñoms*, Orgyan's *'Khrul gcod*, and especially Phadampa Sangye's *Zi byed*.[22] The practice is traditionally linked with the Prajñāpāramitā tradition, wherein the offering of one's body to sentient beings is extolled as an ideal practice of the perfection of generosity (Skt: *dāna pāramitā*). The practice generally features Vajrayoginī or another female deity or *ḍākinī*, and is especially practiced by laywomen and nuns. Codified by the Tibetan *yoginī* Machig Labdron (*Ma gcig lab kyi sgron ma*, 1055–1143), *chö* is a method for severing the tendency to cling to the body and the illusion of self:[23]

> Through offering up one's body—the focal point of physical attachments—one undermines the tendency to reify such dichotomies as subject and object, self and others, and conventional ideas of good and evil. Thus one recognizes that one's fears are only the result of mental afflictions, which themselves are empty of inherent existence. In order to confront them directly, a *chö* practitioner enacts a complex drama consisting of visualizations, rituals, and prayers in which deities and demons are initially conjured up, but later found to be insubstantial, utterly lacking inherent existence, and products of the mind.[24]

Machig's birth narrative recounts her previous life as a *brahmin* dialectician in India. Advised by a *ḍākinī* to flee his opponents, the purified consciousness abandoned the male *brahmin* body in a cave near Vārāṇasī and took birth as Machig in Tibet. From early childhood, Machig gained renown as a *yoginī* and eventually became the progenitor of the deconstructionist *chö* rite. As John Powers notes, she "holds the distinction of being the only Tibetan lama whose teachings were transmitted to India."[25]

The *chö* ritual that Machig disseminated became a popular practice in Tibet that dealt with death in a very profound and immediate way. It incorporated many teachings simultaneously: compassion, emptiness, the sufferings of the six realms, the constructed nature of the self, and the tenuous nature of the body that disintegrates at death. Gaining familiarity with the insubstantial nature of the visualizations leads to direct insight into the ultimately insubstantial nature of conventional reality, cutting through attachments to the body and the self.

Guru, Deity, and Self

The tantric path speaks about one's mind becoming inseparable from the mind of the *guru* and the meditational deity. In the orthodox

Buddhist context this is not possible, since each individuated mental continuum evolves independently toward its own liberation or enlightenment. Individual mind streams do not simply conjoin. The statement that "one's mind becomes inseparable from the mind of the *guru*" therefore represents a conundrum. The most common interpretation is figurative: one's mind becomes enlightened just like the mind of the *guru*. Because the mind is by nature empty, all sentient beings have Buddha nature, the potential for enlightenment. Because one's mind is empty by nature, one can realize the *guru*'s enlightened state.

The tantric meditations use procreative metaphors to symbolize transformation: the divine conjugal couple as the parents, the *maṇḍala* of the deity as the environment, the womb as the genetrix, and the practitioner's mind as the embryo of enlightenment.[26] The tantric meditations also speak about "generating the pride of being the deity," that is, pride in the visualization of oneself as inseparable from the meditational deity (*yidam*): Avalokiteśvara, Mañjuśrī, Vajrapāṇi, Tārā, and others. This identification of oneself with a meditational deity—selected from an infinite number of different manifestations of enlightenment—is not merely symbolic. One takes pride in actually "being" the deity, manifesting all that being's enlightened qualities: compassion, wisdom, power, enlightened activity, and so forth. Since enlightened beings are also individual, each one being the result of a long process of evolution, the identification of the practitioner with the deity is similarly problematic. In order to be consistent with the Mahāyāna hermeneutical framework, the identification must, again, be taken figuratively, that is, by juxtaposing the obscured mental continuum of the ordinary being and the unobscured awareness of the enlightened being.

Madhyamaka: The Perfect View

The Madhyamaka doctrine that came to predominate in Tibet was grounded in the thought of Nāgārjuna, who expounded two levels of truth: conventional and ultimate. He taught that the self exists conventionally and functions on the everyday level of reality, but is ultimately empty—devoid of true existence. These two levels of truth are not regarded as contradictory, but complementary and mutually entailing:

> How could those—that themselves
> Exist individually—be mutually dependent?
> How could those—that do not themselves
> Exist individually—be mutually dependent?[27]

This mode of analysis is applied to all the constituents of the self and similarly to all phenomena. Death and the persons who die also exist conventionally, at an everyday level of reality, but ultimately lack true existence. Why fear the extinction at death of what ultimately has no existence?

As long as the aggregates are conceived to truly exist, the self is also conceived to truly exist; on the basis of this misconception, actions are committed that cause beings to spin within cyclic existence (*saṃsāra*), and experience the sufferings of birth, sickness, old age, and death. When beings achieve the wisdom understanding emptiness, they gain insight into the empty nature of the aggregates and the self, and stop creating actions that give rise to the sufferings of cyclic existence. Nāgārjuna explains:

> Because this wheel is not obtained from self, other
> Or from both, in the past, the present, or the future,
> The conception of I is overcome
> And thereby action and rebirth.[28]

When one uproots the misconception of a truly existent self—arising from itself, another, or both, in the past, present, or future—all other delusions are uprooted automatically.

What becomes of the emptiness of the person at the time of death? The conventional nature of the person (the everyday self) and the ultimate nature of the person (emptiness) are equally empty, and their empty nature is what makes transformation possible. Emptiness in Prāsaṅgika Madhyamaka is always relative to a specific referent. Each phenomenon has its specific emptiness: the emptiness of the vase, the emptiness of the self, the emptiness of emptiness. Interpreters of emptiness must always answer the question, empty of what? Emptiness in the Prāsaṅgika system refers very specifically to the lack of inherent existence of phenomena and not to any entity. Emptiness is the lack of inherent existence of phenomena and there is no emptiness apart from phenomena. Each phenomenon has its specific emptiness (lack of inherent existence), so when the phenomenon disintegrates, its emptiness ceases, also. The emptiness of the vase refers to the vase's lack of inherent existence, so when the vase ceases to exist, its emptiness, or lack of inherent existence, also ceases to exist along with it. Correspondingly, when the person ceases at death, the emptiness of the person ceases as well.

Tibetan Interpretations of Yogācāra Thought

The Prāsaṅgika Madhyamaka system eventually became dominant in Tibet, though Yogācāra views were influencial during the early transmission of Buddhism to Tibet and are prevalent among Tibetan practitioners even today. Tibetan scholars study Asaṅga and Vasubandhu, but the Prāsaṅgika Madhyamaka perspective is the preferred view among scholars at the Tibetan monastic universities. The Yogācāra and Madyamaka perspectives are explained as examples of the Buddha's expedient means (upāya), addressed to individuals of varying capacities. Occasionally the two systems of thought are even explained in tandem. According to Śāntarakṣita, the great Indian pandit who traveled to Tibet in the eighth century, the mind-only view (vijñānamātra) of Yogācāra is useful for understanding conventional reality (all things proceed from the mind), yet the mind (vijñāna) itself lacks own-being.[29] Also, Madhyamaka interpretations often predominate in the philosophical context, while Yogācāra interpretations are influential in the tantric context.

Tibetan Buddhist commentaries are full of debates and polemics between adherents of the Madhyamaka and Yogācāra schools. Madhyamaka proponents critique the Yogācāra theory that all phenomena exist only as they appear to the mind as inadequate to explain conventional realities and as incompatible with lived experience. Madhyamaka followers concede that all experience is ultimately mentally created, in the sense that, out of ignorance and other delusions, we create actions that result in pleasant and unpleasant experiences. The claim that all experience is ultimately mentally created is not the same as the claim that only consciousness exists, however. All waking experience is a product of the mind insofar as phenomena are objects of awareness and actions arise from volitions of the mind, but that is not to say that external objects do not exist at all. By contrast, in the Yogācāra view, all phenomena are said to exist, not externally, but only as they appear to the mind. These two different epistemological claims lead to different views of self-identity and death.

Proponents of the Prāsaṅgika Madhyamaka school interpret tathāgatagarbha as the empty nature of the mind. Being empty of inherent existence, the mind of each sentient being has the potential to achieve the perfect enlightenment of a Buddha. They reason that if the mental continuum were inherently existent, it would be static and therefore impervious to change or evolution. Because the tathāgatagarbha does not have inherent existence and is therefore not static, it is capable of transforming from a deluded state to the enlightened state of awareness that constitutes Buddhahood. Similarly, because the mental continuum is empty and not fixed, change is possible and therefore it is possible for the mental continuum to evolve from a totally obscured state to a perfectly awakened state. The tathāgatagarbha cannot be equated with dharmakāya, however, for although both are empty by nature, the potential to become enlightened is not equivalent to the state of perfect enlightenment, just as a seed is not the same as its resultant sprout. The *tathāgatagarbha* is not the *ālayavijñāna*, nor is it the ground of *saṃsāra* and *nirvāṇa*, for there is no ground of *saṃsāra* and *nirvāṇa*. Both *tathāgatagarbha* and *dharmakāya*, *saṃsāra* and *nirvāṇa* are empty by nature, as are all phenomena whatsoever, but this fact does not erase conventional phenomenological distinctions. To erase phenomenological distinctions on the basis of the empty nature of phenomena leads to the absurd conclusion that all phenomena are indistinguishable, which is contrary to observable reality. The Prāsaṅgika reasoning rests on the premise that emptiness is not a monolithic concept, but simply the absence of inherent existence of all specific phenomena.

A Madhyamaka Critique of Yogācāra Thought

As in early Buddhist thought, the Madhyamaka texts describe six conciousnesses. They do not admit the existence of the additional three consciousnesses that appear in the Yogācāra texts: storehouse consciousness (*ālayavijñāna*), deluded consciousness (*manovijñāna*), or purified consciousness (*amalavijñāna*). Neither do they posit a faculty of self-awareness, a consciousness that is aware of itself (*svasaṃvedanā*). Instead, mental consciousness itself has the capacity to understand its own true nature and its own processes, without the need for a separate self-reflective mechanism. The mental consciousness simply knows, because knowing is its nature. Precisely because the mental consciousness has the capacity to know, perception (direct and inferential, conceptual and nonconceptual) is possible. The superimposition of conceptual structures upon experience creates a distance between the perceiver and direct perception, and the perceiver's direct awareness of the object of awareness becomes obscured and distorted by this conceptual overlay. By eliminating this conceptual overlay through cultivating direct awareness, it is possible to know the true nature of the mind and the self, as well as all other phenomena. Additional conceptual constructs such as self-reflective awareness are superfluous. But the true nature of the mind and the true nature of the self are two separate subjects, or rather, separate objects of perception, even though both are empty by nature. The equation of mind and self that is an easy conceptual leap from a Yogācāra standpoint, is an impossibility in Madhyamaka.

Madhyamaka texts do not posit the existence of a storehouse consciousness *ālayavijñāna* because an additional consciousness is not necessary for storing the predispositions or imprints (*vāsanā*) of actions. The mental continuum itself stores these impressions; in fact, it might be argued that, apart from "knowing," or direct perception, storing the "seeds" of actions is a primary function of mental consciousness. The momentary mental continuum is itself adequate to the task of relaying the imprints of actions without positing an *ālayavijñāna*. In fact, positing an *ālayavijñāna* is risky in that it may be mistaken for a substratum of self or consciousness.

By the same logic, the concept of *manovijñāna*, a deluded consciousness posited by the Yogācāra is also unnecessary and risky. Deluded consciousnesses are merely moments of mental consciousness that are obscured by delusions such as greed, hatred, and ignorance. A separate, deluded consciousness such as the *manovijñāna* that is defiled by nature, if it were to exist, would be a consciousness that cannot be purified. Not only does this raise questions about the relationship of such a consciousness to the mental consciousness, but such a consciousness can also be mistaken for a substratum of self or consciousness that permanently exists, and is thus not consistent with orthodox Buddhist theory. In traditional exegesis, consciousness is impermanent and therefore there is no instance of consciousness, however deluded, that cannot be purified.

In addition to *ālayavijñāna* and *manovijñāna*, the sixth-century Indian monk Paramārtha posits a purified consciousness (*amalavijñāna*) that exists apart from mental consciousness itself. Purified consciousness is described as nothing other than consciousness purified of delusions. But according to Madhyamaka theory, there is no need to posit a separate purified consciousness that exists apart from and simultaneously with ordinary consciousness. Mental consciousness itself, being impermanent, can be purified. As soon as delusion and the stains of delusion are eradicated, enlightened awareness (Buddhahood) is automatically attained. No purified consciousness exists apart from and simultaneous with an individual's ordinary consciousness; if an individual's mental consciousness is totally purified, the being has already achieved Buddhahood. Paramārtha's purified consciousness (*amalavijñāna*) is therefore shown to be an unnecessary superimposition, and one that can easily be mistaken for a substratum of self or consciousness, as *tathāgatagarbha* commonly is. This interpretation is not consistent with orthodox Buddhist theory.

Tibetan commentaries explain *tathāgatagarbha* as the ultimately empty (*śūnya*) nature of the mind, which is what enables the ordinary deluded consciousness to become transformed into enlightened awareness. The Tibetan view of *tathāgatagarbha* is based primarily on three texts attributed to Maitreya as transmitted to Asaṅga: *Sūtrālanakara* (*Ornament for the Mahāyāna Sūtras*), *Uttaratantra* (*Sublime Continuum of the Mahāyāna*), and *Abhisamayālankara* (*Ornament for Clear Realization*). The first describes the natural potential that is the basis for developing the enlightened qualities of a Buddha. The second describes the clear light nature of the mind and the nine analogies used to explain the *tathāgatagarbha*, or potential for enlightenment: (1) the lotus that grows stainless from the mud; (2) bees that expertly extract honey from flowers; (3) the husk that covers grain; (4) a filthy swamp that obscures gold; (5) earth that conceals a treasure; (6) the seed of the mango (and other) fruit; (7) tattered cloth that covers an exquisite Buddha statue; (8) a womb that holds a great future king; and (9) a clay mould that encases a gold Buddha statue. In each case, the analogy points to a pure substance temporarily covered and emerging from something impure.[30] Nevertheless, the *tathāgatagarbha* illustrated by these images is definitely a potentiality, rather than manifest enlightenment. As a potentiality, the concept of *tathāgatagarbha* is clearly independent of an *ālayavijñāna*.

Tibetan scholars continue a tradition of distinguishing two streams of Yogācāra thought: one that "follows scripture," namely, the writings of Asaṅga, and one that "follows reasoning," namely, the reasoning of Dignāga. In the latter stream, the *ālayavijñāna* is viewed as similar to a hibernating consciousness. This view explains how a *yogi*'s awareness can reanimate after a state of deep trance or how a bear upon awakening from hibernation remembers being bitten by a marmot. Gradually this consciousness becomes associated with the subtle consciousness that continues beyond death. "Once the *ālaya-vijñāna* has become associated with the subtle consciousness present at the moment of conception," as Graham Sparham notes, "it was but a short step to the notion that the *ālaya-vijñāna* was the basic constituent of personality."[31] Even though the *ālayavijñāna* is a momentary, composite phenomenon, in certain Tibetan sub-schools it begins to resemble a structure to support the notion of a self or independent identity:

The *ālaya-vijñāna* presented itself as a perfect solution to this perennial problem [of what transmigrates]. As perhaps the deepest subconscious element, the one which was first on the scene and last off, so to speak, during a lifetime, it was to all intents and purposes a constant within the everchanging flux of the psychophysical constituents and eminently suited to function as a soul without actually being one.[32]

The fourteenth-century Tibetan scholar Tsongkhapa rejects this convenient paradigm in no uncertain terms. He traces the evolution of a sentient being through the *bardo* to conception, and hence to luminosity (*prabhāsvara*) at the time of death without any need for an *ālaya-vijñāna* in the process of awakening. He explains how, through Buddhist *tantra*, the experience of the clear light is simulated in meditation practice and then integrated at the time of death for actualizing the *dharmakāya*, or fully awakened state:

> Using the metaphor of child and mother (the same person but at different periods), Tsong kha pa says that "child luminosity" (Tib. *bu 'od gsal*) is the content of the visionary experience before death that is the outcome of a long cultivation of the ultimate truth realized in a properly graduated course of study. Through meditation it becomes an integrated experience. When integrated, it is "mother luminosity" (Tib. *ma'i 'od gsal*), the actual death experience, and becomes, through the process of recognition, part of a natural process such that one realizes the Dharma-kāya ("Truth Body") and remains in an enlightened state.[33]

Tsongkhapa refutes the Yogācāra definition of emptiness as the non-duality of subject and object, citing Candrakīrti's explication in the *Madhyamakāvatāra*. Although the ontological status of knower and known are identical—existing conventionally, but ultimately empty of inherent existence—this is very different than asserting the identity of knower and known.

These contrasts between the Yogācāra and Madhyamaka approaches are reflected in very different cultural practices at the time of death. Pure Land practice in the Tibetan tradition was generally based on Madhyamaka rather than Yogācāra philosophical foundations. In place of an *ālayavijñāna*, there was simply consciousness. Instead of the subjective idealism of Yogācāra, the radical deconstructionist approach of the Madhyamaka prevailed. Instead of being transported to Sukhāvavatī Pure Land by the grace of Amitābha Buddha after death, a person's body is fed to the birds after the dying person has carefully negotiated the process of his or her own physical and psychological dissolution.

Chapter 7

The Transition Between Life and Death

The ultimate objective for Buddhists is the attainment of liberation from the wheel of rebirth, for unless liberation is reached, the sufferings and dissatisfactions of *saṃsāra* continue indefinitely. Unless an individual conscientiously attempts to purify his or her mental continuum of defilements like greed, hatred, and ignorance, these impressions produced by former actions will continue to be transmitted throughout successive lifetimes, repeating themselves over and over. This understanding of cyclic existence is the foundation of all Buddhist practices and therefore the texts and commentaries of all Buddhist traditions have a great deal to say about the nature of death and dying. But it is the Tibetan texts and commentaries that have the most to say about what is experienced during the transition between death of the physical body and the next rebirth. These texts provide instructions for understanding the mechanics of the dying process as well as for negotiating the journey. From them, we learn that death is not a final destination, but simply one momentary event in a succession of moments of transition from one existence to another. This realization frees us from conventional expectations and allows us to experience dying on its own terms.

The relationship between life, death, the *bardo* state, and rebirth is so subtle and complex that it is not easily grasped by the ordinary mind. The link between a person's identity in this lifetime and the next is as tenuous as the thread of connectedness between one moment of consciousness and the next. As real as our self-identity may appear to us in our ordinary, unawakened state, the elements that constitute that identity are not concrete, but ephemeral, each dependent on the causal relationships connecting one moment and the next. The tendency to grasp at individual identity results from misconceiving the self as substantial and enduring. This gives rise to many problems, both in everyday life and at the end of life. Although the ordinary tendency to grasp at an inaccurate concept of self is natural, it also gives rise to the fear and depression that accompany illness and explains, in part, why a terminal diagnosis comes as such a terrible shock. For Buddhists, correcting misconceptions about the nature of the self is central to eliminating the anxiety and suffering that complicate the experience of dying and rebirth. Insight into the connections between lifetimes, and the way our actions and their consequences affect this process puts us in a much better position to skillfully navigate the journey.

Whereas dying is the process during which the physical and mental components of an individual disintegrate, death is the culmination of this process. When the physical body is no longer capable of sustaining life, the coarser states of consciousness disintegrate, one after the other, leaving only the continuity of a very subtle level of consciousness. What happens after that is a matter of interpretation among the different Buddhist schools. A diverse range of viewpoints are presented in the Buddhist texts, and different Buddhist traditions further vary in their practical applications of the ideas presented in these texts. In this chapter, I will discuss these different perspectives and the relevance they have for a cross-cultural dialogue on bioethics. First, I trace the roots of the *bardo* concept to its Indian sources and discuss its variant interpretations. Next, I explain Tibetan interpretations in more detail. Finally, I explore why an understanding of the *bardo* concept may be helpful for facilitating a smooth transition from death to rebirth and why it is relevant to a discussion of liberation, enlightenment, and end-of-life decision making.

Indian Buddhist Concepts of the Intermediate State

The idea of an intermediate state (*antarābhava*, Tib: *bardo*) has its precursors in classical Indian thought. As Arindam Chakrabarti points out, all philosophical schools agree that death is but "a change of phase in the continuing story of the life of a single individual, even if that individual is reducible to a causally connected set and series of psychophysical states)."[1] Vedic eschatology described several distinct "paths" after death: (1) the "ancestral" path (*pitṛyāna*); (2) the illuminated path of the gods (*devayānam*); and (3) immediate rebirth as an insect or other subhuman state without any interlude. The ancestral path, achieved through the performance of rituals and duties, entails a lengthy journey though a dark liminal state, culminating in a human rebirth. The path of the gods, achieved through renunciation and worship of God, entails a lengthy journey through a bright liminal state, culminating in rebirth among the gods.[2] In this formulation, the nature of consciousness is clearly distinguished from the nature of the body.

The existence of an intermediate state between death and rebirth was rejected by the early Buddhist schools (*nikāyas*), including the Theravāda, Vibhajyavādin, Mahāsaṅghika, early Mahīśāsakā, and Dharmaguptaka, and therefore Indian literary sources discussing the concept are few.[3] According to these schools, rebirth occurs immediately after death:

> This last moment of consciousness before death is known as the *cuti viññāna*. Immediately on its cessation, contingent upon some *kamma*, conditioned by the *cuti viññāna*, and driven by craving and ignorance not yet abandoned, there arises in the mother's womb the first stirring of consciousness of the succeeding birth. It is known as the rebirth-linking consciousness (*paṭisandhi viññāna*).[4]

In the *Mahātanhāsaṅkhayasutta*, there is mention of the *gandharva* (smell eater) "about to enter the womb" (*tatrūpakasatta*) or "ready to exist" (*paccupaṭṭhito hoti*), but Buddhaghoṣa insists that this is not an *antarābhava* (intermediate being).[5] The Sarvāstivāda, Vātsīputrīya, Sammatīya, Pūvaśaila, later Mahīśāsakā, and Dārṣṭantika schools accepted the idea of an *antarābhava*.[6]

The concept of *bhavaṅga* (becoming or becomingness), was presumably formulated to explain how the effects of actions are transmitted to future lives without sacrificing the doctrine of momentariness. *Bhavaṅga* first appeared in the early Abhidharma literature. According to Peter Harvey, however, the concept of "becoming," a state between lives in which a non-returner attains *nirvāṇa*, appears in the early *sūtras*.[7] The term *bhavaṅga* is interpreted either as an "unconscious continuum" or a factor that links *karma* to future rebirths. Harvey suggests that it was "both a vehicle for transferring the continuity of character and also a time for the necessary re-adjustment" between disparate forms of rebirth.[8] An "essentially passive state,"[9] the *bhavaṅga* state seems to be the basis upon which the concept of *ālayavijñāna* (storehouse consciousness) eventually develops. The *gandharva* concept persists in the minds of many Theravāda Buddhists up to the present day, taking on a spirit-like existence, but there is also considerable resistance to it on the part of scholars, who presumably fear it be construed as a "transmigrating personality."[10]

In early Mahāyāna sources, the best sources of information about the *antarābhava* are Vasubandhu's *Abhidharmakośa* and its autocommentary, the *Abhidharmakośabhāsyam*.[11] In these texts, Vasubandhu explains the concept of *antarābhava* as one of seven existences (*bhava*).[12] Citing references to the concept of *gandharva*[13] in the early *sūtras*,[14] he interprets *antarābhava* as "one who attains *nirvāṇa* in the intermediate state." Instead of interpreting the concept *antarāparinirvāyin* as one of five types of non-returner (*anāgāmin*) beings, he explains it as one who attains *nirvāṇa* in a god realm.[15] Except for those who take rebirth in the hells as a result of having committed one of the five heinous crimes (*ānantarya*),[16] in which case retribution occurs immediately after death, an intermediate state "arises" (*upapadyamāna*) because the intermediate "being" is inclined toward its next birth (*upapatti*).[17]

According to Vasubandhu, a *bardo* being takes a form that presages the existence it will take in the next rebirth. That is to say, the form a being takes in the intermediate state between death and conception prefigures the being's future rebirth. For example, if the *bardo* being has created actions (*karma*) that will result in a rebirth as a human being (or a dog or a heavenly being), that being will take an intermediate existence in that form, prior to taking rebirth as that particular type of being. This makes sense, since the form a being takes in the *bardo* is a result of the same type of actions that will propel the being to take that same form of identity in its next rebirth (*pūrvakālabhava*).[18] The intermediate being seeks a suitable rebirth and, if one is not found within seven days, experiences a "small death" and then another *bardo* "birth." This process may be repeated up to seven times, after which time conception must take place. Here, the intermediate state refers only to the period between death and conception, not to the period of intra-uterine development.

The form that the intermediate being takes is intangible and invisible to the ordinary eye. In seeking a suitable rebirth, the *bardo* being is able to travel without being obstructed by walls or any other material barriers. The *bardo* being, variously known as *gandharva* (smell eater) and *manomaya* (made of mind), is visible only to similar types of beings and to those who have achieved the divine eye through higher knowledge, or paranormal perception (*atikrānta-mānusyaka*). Despite lacking the physical sense organs, such a being has the six sense bases (*ṣaḍāyatana*) and therefore the capacity for sense perceptions. Each *bardo* existence lasts for a maximum of seven days, after which the *bardo* being must take another rebirth. If a suitable rebirth is not found (i.e., the complex matrix of causes necessary for rebirth has not been realized), a *bardo* being can take up to seven intermediate existences, each seven days in length, up to a total of forty-nine days, after which time that being must take the next rebirth. When the *bardo* being finds suitable conditions (a healthy womb and parents in coitus), it enters the mother's womb, the intermediate state ends, and the next life begins. Beings destined for the formless realm (*ārūpadhātu*) do not experience any intermediate state. The *Mārasūtra* mentions the case of a *māra* named Dūṣin who, because of his grave transgressions, was reborn immediately in hell without any intermediate (*antarā*) dwelling (*vāsa*).[19] This case can be construed to mean that individuals who have created seriously unwholesome actions are deprived of the opportunities presented in the intermediate state, whereas those who have created wholesome actions have earned those opportunities.

Tibetan Ways of Dying Mindfully

The Tibetan Buddhist tradition has developed a panoplay of methods for mental cultivation that help human beings to live more consciously and also help them prepare for dying. By training in a range of methods of mental cultivation (*bhāvana*), practitioners gain an understanding of the different types of conscious awareness and, through disciplined practice, become better able to control them. Eventually practitioners learn to distinguish between coarser and more subtle states of consciousness, and they develop greater awareness of the relationship between the mind and the body. Proficiency in understanding how the different types of consciousness function and learning how to control them is closely linked to the process of accumulating merit and wisdom toward the goal of awakening, and is especially useful during the dying process. For this reason, the experience of dying is simulated and rehearsed during meditation practice. Learning to recognize the basic "clear and knowing" nature of the mind enables a practitioner to understand the true nature of the mind, an insight that is helpful for contented and meaningful living, but also, perhaps more importantly, while dying. According to Tibetan sources, understanding the true nature of the mind is also of crucial importance during the journey between life, death, and rebirth.

Tibetan epistemology postulates an intimate relationship between consciousness and the sense faculties and between consciousness and actions created (*karma*). It further postulates that consciousness functions on several levels. The coarser levels of consciousness are generated as a result of contact between a physical sense base and its object; more subtle levels of consciousness are generated in relation to the mental sense base and may operate independently of the body. These subtle levels of consciousness are elucidated in detail in various tantric texts. The Dalai Lama explains the nature of mind as presented in this system:

> According to tantra, the ultimate nature of mind is essentially pure. This pristine nature is technically called "clear light." The various afflictive emotions such as desire, hatred and jealousy are products of conditioning. They are not intrinsic qualities of the mind because the mind can be cleansed of them.[20]

That mind has the nature of light is a notion not confined only to the tantric texts; early Buddhist schools also portray the nature of consciousness (*citta*) as "brightly shining."[21] Peter Harvey describes how the light imagery was taken up and expanded in the Mahāyāna tradition:

> The uncovered brightly shining *citta* is thus the ideal springboard from which to attain awakening, such that it can be seen as a kind of enlightenment-potential. Appropriately, one strand of Mahāyāna thought identifies the brightly shining *citta* with the *tathāgata-garbha*.[22]

The *Laṅkavātāra Sūtra* takes this metaphor further when it associates the brightly shining nature of the *tathāgatagarbha* with original purity. The clear light of death mentioned in Tibetan tantric texts occurs just after death, and before the *bardo* begins. If that is the case, theoretically at least, it is possible that liberation arising from a recognition of the clear light may occur even among those who reject the *bardo* concept.

The preliminaries for conscious dying begin with a series of reflections on the nature of death, its implications, and its inevitability.[23] Meditating on death, one first reflects on the fact that death is definite, by considering that: (1) death comes to everyone; (2) one's life span is constantly diminishing and cannot be extended indefinitely; and (3) while one is alive, little time is spent on mental cultivation. In the second part of the meditation, one reflects on the fact that the time of death is indefinite, by considering that: (1) the human life span is not fixed; (2) the causes of death are many and the conditions for supporting life are few; and (3) the human body is very fragile. In the last part of the meditation, one reflects on the fact that at the time of death, only mental cultivation is of benefit, by considering that: (1) friends and relatives are of no further use; (2) possessions are of no further use; and (3) one's body is of no further use. Serious reflection on these topics can motivate a person to abandon worldly concerns and concentrate intensively on spiritual practice.

Another method of meditating on death is to visualize the dissolution of the elements of the body and mind that occurs during the stages of dying.[24] The dissolution of the physical and mental elements (earth, water, fire, wind, and consciousness) occurs in conjunction with the dissolution of the five aggregates, accompanied by specific physical, external, and internal signs.[25] For example, the form aggregate is associated with the earth element. As the form aggregate "dissolves," the most solid constituents of the body (bones, teeth, and nails) begin to disintegrate. On the physical level, the body feels weak and heavy. Internally, one feels depressed and a mirage-like image appears. In this way, a practitioner meditates on each of the signs that appear as the subsequent elements dissolve in sequence: water, fire, and wind. Next, consciousness dissolves in three stages, known as the consciousness of white appearance, the consciousness of red increase, and the consciousness of black appearance. As the consciousness of black appearance dissolves, the clear light of death appears. The luminous refractions in rainbow colors represent the six realms of rebirth: white for the god realm, green for the demi-god realm, yellow for the human realm, blue for the animal realm, red for the hungry ghost realm, and black for the hell realm. At this point, unless a being has purified the mind and overcome all defilements, the consciousness takes another rebirth, impelled by habitual patterns of desire and attachment.

The *bardo* may last from an instant to forty-nine days, depending on the person and the circumstances. In the case of a sudden death, the dissolution of the five elements occurs quickly and the consciousness may take another rebirth immediately. (Some texts speak of six elements—earth, water, fire, wind, ether, and consciousness.) When an ordinary, unenlightened person dies a natural death, the *bardo* experience usually lasts from one to three days. Tibetans typically request a divination from a respected *lama* to determine the appropriate time for disposing of the corpse, to ensure that the person's consciousness has already departed from the body, and to determine which prayers and rituals will most benefit the deceased.

For a serious Buddhist practitioner, the *bardo* may last longer than just a few days. A person who has practiced well and purified mental defilements may remain conscious during the dissolution of the elements and achieve enlightenment by recognizing the clear light nature of the mind during the *bardo*. There are reported cases of practitioners who remained in a state of meditation for several days after the heartbeat and breathing ceased, with discernible warmth in the heart region and without decomposing. The twenty-sixth Gyalwa Karmapa and Kyabje Ling Rinpoche, the senior tutor of the present Dalai Lama, both of whom passed away in 1982, are examples.[26] Even people who appear quite ordinary are sometimes able to achieve this. The remains (*sku gdung*) of such master practitioners often become objects of veneration.

One who has not practiced and is not familiar with the stages of the dying process may experience terrifying visions and sensations during the intermediate state. Even those who are not serious practitioners are advised to familiarize themselves with the stages of dying in order to dispel fear and despair, and avoid the mental suffering that can accompany the dissolution of the physical elements. In the Tibetan Buddhist *bardo* literature, it is said that as the earth element dissolves, there is a sensation of being trampled by herds of animals. As the water element dissolves, it is like falling into a turbulent ocean. As the fire element dissolves, it is like being burnt in a bonfire. And as the wind element dissolves, it is like being thrashed by a fierce wind. The terror that the dying person might experience as a result of these sensations can be mitigated by Dharma practice, by gaining familiarity in advance with the types of visions and sensations that accompany the dissolution of the elements. For example, instead of feeling thrashed by a fierce gale as the wind element dissolves, one can experience the wind as a gentle breeze.

Equally as important, one practices in order to become aware of the successive patent signs of dying as they transpire. One learns to recognize the white drop that descends from the forehead to the heart, the red drop that ascends from the navel to the heart, and the convergence of the two as they join together to enclose the consciousness ("like a tent") at the heart. Death occurs when this tent collapses, at which point the dying person loses consciousness. At this moment, a white substance may be emitted from the right nostril and a drop of blood from the left.[27] These signs are sometimes observed by medical attendants of the dying, especially if they are trained to be aware of these indicators of passage. In certain cases, skilled practitioners may be able to maintain awareness of the convergence of the consciousness in this "tent" for a year or more. Cases such as those of the Sixth Panchen Lama, who died in 1935, and Je Khenpo, the recent chief abbot of Bhutan who died in 1999, have been observed by many people.[28] Experienced practitioners such as these are said to remain in a state of *samādhi*, during which time, unencumbered by the ordinary distractions of life and physical functions, they are able to make rapid progress toward enlightenment. To be on the safe side, Buddhist families of means often continue to perform prayers and rituals for their loved ones for a full forty-nine days, even if they were ordinary individuals.

During the intermediate state, the aim is to be completely aware when the actual moment of death occurs and to be able to recognize the clear light nature of consciousness when it appears. Without fear or distraction, the skilled meditator is able to directly realize the clear light as being empty (*sūnya*) by nature. The process of purification and attunement that occurs when one remains fully alert and continuously mindful of the clear light nature of the mind during the *bardo* is an opportunity for successive levels of realization, even liberation. Just like during the dream state between sleep and wakefulness, known as the intermediate dream state (*rmi lam bar do*), the subtle consciousness continues. Because the experience of the clear light is an opportunity to recognize the "indivisibility of motility and mentality," the constantly changing nature of consciousness, Guenther calls it an "intermediate state of possibilities."[29] It is not that these subtle states of consciousness are not present during ordinary waking life; it is just that most people are so absorbed with coarser levels of consciousness that they live their lives unaware of the more subtle states.

However, as the physical body disintegrates, the coarser levels of consciousness gradually also disintegrate and have less impact on a person's awareness. For this reason, the states of the dying process provide an enhanced opportunity to become more receptive or tuned in, and therefore more cognizant of these subtle levels of consciousness. Unfortunately, unless the dying person is familiar with these more subtle levels of consciousness through having engaged in intensive meditation practice on the stages of dying, the person will be unable to recognize and take advantage of the opportunities that present themselves during the intermediate state. Oblivious of the true clear light nature of consciousness and of the brilliant opportunities for achieving realization and enlightenment that arise only during the intermediate state, the chance of a lifetime will be wasted.

Personal Identity in the Afterdeath State

According to Bryan J. Cuevas' historical overview of the *bardo* concept, the *antarābhava* concept originally appears in the Abhidharma literature, especially in the literature of the Sarvāstivāda school, which specifically refers to an intermediate state between death and rebirth.[30]

In the *Abhidharmakośabhāsyam*, Vasubhandu refers to the *antarābhava* in three contexts: the *Saptabhavasūtra* mentions it as one of seven possible existences (*bhava*); the *Āśvalāyanasūtra* regards it as an incipient being;[31] and various texts in the Pāli canon explain it as one type of *anāgāmin* (non-returner):

> The Blessed One teaches that there are five types of Anā-gāmins: one who obtains Nirvāṇa in an intermediate existence (*antarāparinirvāyin*), one who obtains Nirvāṇa as soon as he is reborn (*upapadyaparinirvāyin*), one who obtains Nirvāṇa without effort (*anabhisaṃskāraparinirvāyin*), one who obtains Nirvāṇa by means of effort (*anabhisaṃskāraparinirvāyin*), and one who obtains Nirvāṇa by going higher (*ūrdvasrotas*).[32]

This passage not only refers to an intermediate state (*antarābhava*) in the Buddha's teachings, but also to the existence of beings who achieve liberation in the intermediate state (*antarāparinirvāyin*). A classification of three types of *antarāparinirvāyin* according to duration and place appears in both Pāli and Sanskrit texts.[33]

In time, the concept of *antarābhava* (Tib: *bardo*) became elaborated into four stages: birth, life, death, and the interval between death and rebirth. Three of these stages gradually became identified with the three bodies (*trikāya*) of a Buddha: *dharmakāya*, *sambhogakāya*, and *nirmanakāya*. By understanding the nature of one's own mind as the union of clear light and emptiness, one recognizes the clear light of death as the *dharmakāya*, or "truth body." By consciously directing the visions and experiences of the intermediate state, one transforms the *bardo* into the *sambhogakāya*, or "enjoyment body." By consciously directing the rebirth process, one transforms birth into the *nirmaṇakāya*, or "emanation body."[34] The synthesis thus represents an integration of the ordinary processes of death, intermediate state, and rebirth with the generation and completion stages of tantric practice. Through the practice of "deity *yoga*," visualizing oneself in the aspect of an enlightened being, one simulates the state of enlightenment. In this way, the adept becomes skilled at closing the door to further rebirth, a practice known as "obstructing the *bardo*." At the same time, the practice of assuming an alternative, enlightened identity undermines the individual's allegiance to accustomed mistaken identifications. By extension, the practice undercuts the individual's customary perceptions of reality *in toto*.

The eleventh-century Indian master Nāropa (1016–1100) innovatively drew correlations between several sets of three. He related life, death, and rebirth to the *trikāya* doctrine, to the three levels of practitioners (dull, medium, and sharp), and to the visions that appear to the dying, in what has become a standard tantric practice formula in the New Translation Schools of Buddhism in Tibet. Nāropa's Tibetan disciple Marpa Lotsawa (*Rje btsun lho brag pa*, 1012–1097) further developed this schema by integrating a threefold taxonomy of the *bardo* into foundation (correct view of emptiness), path (practice method), and fruit (attainment of enlightenment). Marpa's disciple Milarepa (*Mi la res pa*, 1040–1123) further elaborated these ideas in *The Song of the Golden Rosary*. Building on Milarepa's ideas and others as well, Yangönpa (*Yang dgon pa*) arrived at a modified list of six *bardos*, namely: (1) the natural state, (2) ripening from birth to death, (3) meditative stabilization, (4) karmic latencies and dreams, (5) dying, and (6) becoming. The ultimate objective of the practice is to utilize the stages in the process of dying and becoming to achieve realization and avoid rebirth. The "*bardo* of reality itself" (*chos nyid bar do*) began to appear in the twelfth century, apparently derived from the Nyingma (*rNying ma*) tradition.

Grasping is said to be the root cause of continual rebirth in cyclic existence. Two types of grasping are elucidated by the Mahāyāna tradition: grasping at persons (the self) and grasping at phenomena as being truly existent, when they are not. To counteract grasping, the Buddha taught the impermanent, painful, illusory nature of self and phenomena. He taught that all phenomena are empty like foam, water bubbles, mirages, echoes, plantain trees, dreams, reflections in a mirror, and conjurers' tricks. Other means of counteracting grasping at personal identity are found in the visualization practices taught in the Vajrayāna tradition. Here, one imagines oneself in the form of an enlightened being (the *yidam*, or meditational deity) in a completely pure realm surrounded by other similarly enlightened beings. This type of visualization practice is taught as a means to cut through the habitual tendency to grasp at the perception of a substantial self. Because it accustoms the individual to a different mode of perception and engenders an awareness of the arbitrary and flexible nature of personal identifications, it is recommended in preparation for death:

> If you gain realization in this practice of the pure body, then during the transitional process following death, it is certain that you will be liberated. It is best if you can be liberated when the peaceful emanations arise and, if not then, when the wrathful appearances arise.[35]

To visualize oneself in the form of a meditational deity removes all fear when the peaceful and wrathful archetypes of enlightened mind appear in the *bardo*. Further, by identifying with the form and enlightened qualities of the deity at all times, one actualizes or "becomes" the deity.[36] Through a process of simulation, one's ordinary identity and environment become transformed into an enlightened identity and pure environment. Ordinary, deluded pride based on self-cherishing and grasping is replaced by the pride of being the deity, based on compassion and the wisdom that directly realizes emptiness. By learning to control the winds of the body and consciously directing them through the psychic channels, a practitioner learns to successfully guide the consciousness at the moment of death to a rebirth in the Pure Land of an enlightened being.

The Profound Dharma of the Natural Liberation through Contemplating the Peaceful and Wrathful: Stage of Completion Instructions on the Six Bardos, a treasure text (ter) attributed to Padmasambhava and discovered by Karma Lingpa (Kar ma gling pa, fourteenth century) names the intermediate states slightly differently than Yangönpa does.[37] It also lists them in a different order, namely, the bardos of (1) living, (2) dreaming, (3) meditative stabilization, (4) dying, (5) reality itself, and (6) becoming. Yangönpa's description of the bardo of the natural state is roughly equivalent to Padmasambhava's bardo of reality itself. The following discussion will consider these six states one by one.

The Bardo of Living

There are four contemplations that are fundamental for subduing one's mind and attaining liberation: (1) the preciousness and rarity of a human rebirth, (2) death and impermanence, (3) the sufferings of cyclic existence, and (4) the law of cause and effect.[38] These are cast as "the four thoughts that turn one's mind to the Dharma." Next, one settles into the posture with seven features, and rests the body, speech, and mind in their natural states.[39] While generating the pure motivation of wishing to achieve awakening for the good of all beings, an unwavering awareness that extends beyond the meditation session into the actions of everyday life is cultivated. Some meditation methods focus on a specific object, while others have no focus, like boundless space. Generally speaking, these approaches are typical of the Gelug (dGe lugs) and Nyingma schools, respectively. The Gelug school presents a gradual approach in which the mind is purified of delusion and eventually transformed into the perfectly enlightened knowing of a Buddha; the Nyingma presents a Chan-like approach in which the mind is regarded as being primordially liberated and the essence of Buddhahood (tathāgatagarbha) is already manifest.[40] Both schools, and the Sakya (Sa skya) and Kagyu (bKa' brgyud) schools as well, turn their attention to meditation on the true nature of the mind itself. According to Gyatrul Rinpoche, a Nyingma lama:

> The awareness in question is simply natural, ordinary aware-
> ness without any type of modification, without any fabrica-
> tion. It is without beginning; it is without birth, remaining,
> or cessation. Failing to recognize its nature, we enter into
> dualistic grasping, grasping onto ourselves, grasping onto
> others, grasping onto our own personal identity, grasping
> onto the identity of other phenomena. In this way we grasp
> onto that which is nonexistent as being existent. As a result
> of that, we continue to wander in the cycle of existence.[41]

This naturally luminous awareness, he says, is "the cause of omni-science." This awareness, as Padmasambhava says, is "inseparable clarity, awareness, and emptiness," "the stainless sole eye of primordial wisdom."[42] In this view, the present human life is *the* most precious window of opportunity for manifesting primordial wisdom. And for those with sharp faculties, there is the potential to manifest omniscient awareness in this very body, in this very life.

The *Bardo* of Dreaming

The instructions on dreaming go hand in hand with the instructions on the illusory body, cultivated through meditation during the daytime. Retreating into solitude and generating an altruistic motivation, one meditates on the mutable, illusory nature of one's body and all other appearances, and how grasping at these binds beings within cyclic existence. On the basis of this practice, called the "pure illusory body," one also trains in the practice of dream yoga. The first step in dream yoga is to begin seeing the phenomena of everyday waking reality, as well as the one perceiving them, as lacking in any essence and thus not different from a dream or an illusion. Next, one goes to bed in the evening and lies in the "lion posture,"[43] while clearly visualizing oneself as one's preferred meditational deity. The immediate aim is to learn to recognize dream states for what they are, in anticipation of apprehending the intermediate state after death for what it is. A series of visualization exercises are employed to sharpen this awareness. For example, during the dream state, one may imagine jumping into a raging river, then experiencing it as bliss and emptiness. Understanding the illusory nature of the phenomena that appear in dreams, one practices transforming them—multiplying, collapsing, and changing them into various shapes and sizes. Progressively, as one continues to practice, a clear recognition of the dream-like, illusory nature of all phenomena and all appearances, waking and sleeping, occurs.

Central to the practice of dream yoga is vivid visualization on the clear light that appears as one falls asleep, until eventually the clear light dawns naturally, clear and empty, during the dream state:

> To apprehend the clear light in the nature of reality-itself, you who nakedly identify awareness should position your body as before, subdue your awareness, and in vivid clarity and emptiness focus your awareness at your heart, and fall asleep. When your sleep is agitated, do not lose the sense of indivisible clarity and emptiness. When you are fast asleep, if the vivid, indivisibly clear and empty light of deep sleep is recognized, the clear light is apprehended.[44]

The clear light appears to all sentient beings at the time of death, but one must be skilled to recognize it for what it is. The clear light also appears at the junctures between wakefulness and sleep, and sleep and wakefulness, but again, one must be skilled in order to glimpse it:[45]

> [The mind of clear light] manifests at periods when the grosser levels of consciousness cease either intentionally, as in profound states of meditation, or naturally, as in the process of death, going to sleep, ending a dream, fainting, and orgasm. Prior to its manifestation, there are several stages during which a practitioner experiences increasingly subtler levels of mind. . . . The winds (or currents of energy; *rlung, prāna*) that serve as foundations for various levels of consciousness are gradually withdrawn, in the process of which one first has a visual experience of seeing an appearance like a mirage . . . billowing smoke . . . fireflies . . . sputtering butter-lamp . . . a steady candle flame. With the withdrawal of conceptual consciousnesses, a more dramatic phase begins, at which point profound levels of consciousness that are at the core of experience manifest.[46]

Even the interval between the cessation of one moment of consciousness and the arising of the next may be an opportunity for glimpsing the clear light.

The identification of one's consciousness with the clear light totally supplants identification with ordinary personal identity. Thus, dream *yoga* is an opportunity to rehearse recognizing the clear light that will appear during the *bardo*. Done well, with perfect wisdom and awareness, the identification of one's consciousness with the clear light will serve as a catalyst for the manifestation of the *dharmakāya*—the perfectly enlightened awareness of the Buddha one becomes. This obviously is the culmination of the practice: the "clear light natural liberation of delusion."[47] One's usual deluded identification is replaced by a thoroughly awakened identification that is beyond the ability of ordinary consciousness to perceive. Whether achieved while awake, asleep, meditating, dreaming, or dying, the *dharmakāya* is at once an evolution of one's ordinary deluded stream of consciousness and an entirely new, omniscient state of awareness.

The *Bardo* of Meditative Stabilization

Among the five aggregates that comprise the Buddhist sense of self-identity, consciousness is unquestionably central. Consciousness, which is synonymous with awareness, is defined as "clear knowing." Thus, according to the teachings of Padmasambhava, to overcome the instinctive grasping at personal identity, it is necessary to relinquish grasping at awareness itself. This can be accomplished through practicing the *bardo* of meditative stabilization.

No matter how profound the teachings or our realizations are, pride and attachment may still remain obstacles to liberation. To prevent pride and attachment from arising, one must go beyond a merely intellectual understanding to a state of direct awareness. Gyatrul Rinpoche comments: "Just as a sword cannot cut itself, and the eye cannot see itself, we have been unable to recognize our own nature."[48] This seems to point to a self-aware consciousness such as is posited by the Yogācāra school, but Padmasambhava does not analyze it as such. In any case, the reference is to the unenlightened, untrained mind. It is through training the mind that one becomes aware of one's own mind. Questions about whether a separate consciousness is required to observe mental consciousness and whether the mind resembles a mirror that sees itself are not questions that concern contemplatives; for them, the goal is to go beyond conceptual thought and, therefore, experience is the only relevant teacher.

The notion of going beyond conceptual thought is not limited to any particular Buddhist school, of course. For example, the rigorously analytical Gelug and Sakya schools acknowledge that direct insight into emptiness is a nonconceptual awareness, that is, a direct awareness that is not dependent upon names and concepts. In these schools, practitioners on the ten *bodhisattva* stages, beginning from the Path of

Insight, meditate until enlightenment by alternating theoretical analysis of emptiness with calm abiding (*śamatha*), using emptiness as the object of meditation. The meditation session begins with a theoretical analysis of emptiness that continues until a very clear realization of emptiness is gained. At that point, the practitioner meditates single-pointedly on emptiness itself until meditative stabilization (*samādhi*) is achieved. When the power of concentration begins to decline after meditating for some time, the practitioner returns to analytical meditation focused on emptiness. In this way, the two practices are alternated—analysis of emptiness and unwavering concentration on emptiness—for the duration of the session. When the meditation session ends, an intellectual understanding of the empty nature of all phenomena is retained, even though ordinary phenomena continue to appear on the conventional level. In the post-meditation state, the practitioner accumulates merit through various other means; direct insight into emptiness (*vipaśyanā*) is achieved primarily through formal meditation practice.

In Tibet, a doctrinal dispute developed between adherents of two different views of emptiness. The *rang tong* (*rang stong*, "self-empty") view, which is prevalent in the more analytical Gelug and Sakya schools, asserts the emptiness of all phenomena, including emptiness, and denies the existence of an absolute reality. The *zhen tong* (*gzhan stong*, "other-empty") view, which is more prevalent in the Kagyu and Nyingma schools, asserts that the "other"—apparent reality—is empty, but there is an ultimate reality (*buddhajñāna*) that truly exists. Adherents of the *rang tong* view interpret *tathāgatagarbha* as the emptiness of inherent existence of the mental continuum that enables sentient beings to achieve enlightenment. The *tathāgatagarbha* was taught for non-Buddhists and needs to be interpreted because, if it were taken literally, it would amount to the same thing as a soul.[49] Adherents of the *zhen tong* view take the *tathāgatagarbha* teachings literally and accept the existence of an ultimate reality that exists inherently.[50] The fact that all beings have the *tathāgatagarbha* means that they have the enlightened awareness of a Buddha, which is just temporarily obscured. When the obscurations are removed, the *dharmakāya* is revealed; therefore, *tathāgatagarbha* and *dharmakāya* are identical. While both approaches aim at nondual, nonconceptual awareness, their philosophical differences, especially their articulations of ultimate truth, have crystallized into what is known as the *rang tong/zhen tong* debate.

The *Bardo* of Dying

For those who have not had time to meditate or are not trained in the practices of the illusory body, dream *yoga*, and the clear light,

Padmasambhava provided instructions on the *bardo* of dying. In the practice of *phowa*, the transference of consciousness, one learns to guide the winds of the body into the central psychic channel, eject the subtle consciousness through the crown *chakra*, and direct it to a Pure Land. The subtle consciousness is not actually ejected until actual death occurs, however, since to do so would cause the practitioner's death and be equivalent to suicide. Therefore it is crucial to ascertain without doubt that death has occurred before actual *phowa* is begun. For a practitioner of deity *yoga*, who practices identification with a *yidam*, to transfer the consciousness prematurely is said to be equivalent to murdering the deity. There are various means of "cheating death"—specific Buddhist practices for longevity such as saving animals' lives and the practices of Amitāyus and White Tārā—that may be attempted. If these are unsuccessful and death becomes certain, one prepares to experience the stages of dying as the physical body and mind disintegrate.[51] When the clear light of death appears, the coarse sense of a self that exists in dependence on the body and mind disintegrates, and a subtle sense of self, imputed to exist in dependence on the subtle energy-mind, takes its place.[52]

The practice of *phowa* (transference of consciousness) begins with a review of the four thoughts that turn one's mind to the Dharma: the precious human rebirth, impermanence, suffering, and the law of cause and effect. After gaining clear insight into the defects of cyclic existence, one develops renunciation—the determination to be liberated from cyclic existence. Sitting in meditation posture, one then visualizes blocking the "apertures of cyclic existence" (anus, genital opening, urinary opening, navel, mouth, nostrils, eyes, and ears), departure through which results in rebirth within the six realms of cyclic existence. One visualizes a central psychic channel extending from below the navel to the crown *chakra* at the top of the head and flanked by subsidiary channels on the right and left. One then concentrates on forcefully drawing the winds and energies of the body up through the central psychic channel along with a radiant white "drop" (*bindu*) in the nature of awareness, and directs them out through the Brahmā aperture at the crown of the head. Except at the time of death, one then visualizes the white drop descending and coming to rest at a point below the navel.

When it becomes clear that actual death is sure to soon occur, it is beneficial to first give away all one's possessions. Whether the generosity is actual or visualized, it creates merit and prevents attachment—the greatest hindrance at the time of death. In fact, objects of attachment or aversion are best removed from a dying person's room, lest they spark unwholesome mental states. Next, one regrets transgressions of the precepts and "restores" them through a ritual confession of faults. Then, sitting in meditation posture, if possible, or in the lion posture, if not, the practice of *phowa* is begun. One reflects:

> Now I am dying. So in general in the three realms of the cycle of existence and in particular in this degenerate era, I rejoice that I can transfer my consciousness while having the companionship of such profound instructions as these. Now I shall recognize the clear light of death as the Dharmakāya, I shall send out immeasurable emanations to train others according to their needs, and I must serve the needs of sentient beings until the cycle of existence is empty.[53]

If the practice of *phowa* is successful, a drop of blood or lymph will appear at the crown of one's head.

If the practice is not successful, one continues through the visualizations, either summoning the visualizations oneself or by having a spiritual mentor or friend recite the instructions in one's ear. If the clear light of death is recognized as inseparable from the clear light nature of the mind (*dharmakāya*), it is possible to become freed from rebirth once and for all, and to achieve either perfect enlightenment or rebirth in a Pure Land where enlightenment can be quickly attained. This is called "the meeting of the mother and child clear light," because it mixes the "mother" clear light of death with the "son" clear light which dawns, through meditation, during sleep and the waking state.[54] If this highest "pristine *dharmakāya* transference of consciousness" is successful, it is confirmed by serene skies and a sustained physical radiance.

If the *dharmakāya* transference is unsuccessful, one attempts the *sambhogakāya* transference. Sitting in meditation posture, if possible, one visualizes the meditational deity at the crown of the head and focuses single-pointedly on a white drop (*bindu*) or seed syllable at the base of the central psychic channel. As in the *phowa* meditation, the vital energies are driven up the central psychic channel to the crown aperture and absorbed into the heart of the meditational deity visualized there. If the transference is successful at death, one becomes a Buddha in *sambhogakāya* form, confirmed by the appearance of deities, rainbows, and relics. If the transference is not successful at the moment of death, one continues the practice during the intermediate state.

If the *sambhogakāya* transference is unsuccessful, one attempts the *nirmāṇakāya* transference. Lying on one's right side, offerings of body, speech, and mind are made to the representation of a Buddha visualized in front of one. Such a visualization helps to break through the possessiveness that arises from strongly identifying with one's ordinary body, speech, and mind. Imagining a red and a white drop in the central psychic channel, one pushes them forcefully upwards until they emerge from the left nostril and dissolve into the heart of the Buddha visualized in front. If the transference is successful and one dies at this point, one becomes a Buddha in *nirmāṇakāya* form, attested by the appearance of clouds and rainbows in auspicious shapes, and flowers falling from the sky. If the body is cremated, the skull remains undamaged. If the transference is not successful at the moment of death, one continues the practice during the intermediate state.

The crown aperture is regarded as the pathway to the Pure Land, whether this be the Pure Land of Amitābha, another Buddha, or the *ḍākinīs* (enlightened energy in female form), and the departure of the consciousness from this aperture signals the achievement of liberation. Departure of the consciousness from the apertures in the upper part of the body is said to lead to fortunate "migrations," while departure from the lower apertures indicates rebirth in unfortunate states. Because one's state of mind, especially at the moment of death, is such a powerful indicator of one's immanent destiny, even beginning practitioners are advised to go for refuge, generate the *bodhicitta*, take precepts, and generate wholesome thoughts as death approaches. After a practitioner has died, a companion may even direct the deceased's attention to a Buddha on the crown of the head, touch the crown, or gently pull the hair at the crown aperture to nudge the consciousness toward a higher realm of rebirth. Reciting the names of the Buddhas (Ratnaśikhin, Amitābha, and so on) and reading the *Liberation Through Hearing* (known as the *Tibetan Book of the Dead*) are also beneficial for helping the person achieve liberation in the *bardo* or a higher rebirth.

The *Bardo* of Reality Itself

The fifth intermediate state, the *bardo* of reality itself, is an opportunity to identify the nature of reality (*dharmatā*) and achieve the natural liberation of seeing. In the Nyingma tradition, this is understood as the practice of Dzogchen, "the Great Perfection." Dzogchen involves prescribed postures and gazes, awareness of the outer and inner "absolute natures" (apprehended as the cloudless sky and a lamp), and learning to hold, expel, and stabilize the vital energies of the body, aimed at realizing primordial wisdom. These practices cause four visions to arise: (1) the direct vision of reality itself, (2) progressing experience, (3) consummate awareness, and (4) extinction into reality itself.[55] Unlike the practices discussed earlier that employ extensive visualizations and recitations, these visions arise independently without ideation. Absolute nature refers to primordial wisdom: clear luminous awareness and emptiness. With practice, *"bindus* of the strand of one's own awareness" appear in the form of primordial wisdom, emanating lights and containing the five divine embodiments of Buddhas with their consorts. Stabilizing a vision of consummate awareness over time, one eventually emanates the *sambhogakāya* effortlessly. The "vision of extinction into reality itself" is the ultimate attainment achieved through the tantric tradition of Dzogchen. Proponents assert that this culminating attainment is higher than what is possible in the *sūtra* tradition, although the descriptions of omniscient Buddhahood (knowing all that is, as it is) are identical in Dzogchen and other tantric traditions.

The *Bardo* of Becoming

The final *bardo*, the *bardo* of becoming, is for those who have not succeeded in any of the preceding five transitional processes and are therefore subject to taking rebirth. After realizing oneself to be dead and wandering in the intermediate state, one visualizes arising in the form of a meditational deity in a pure Buddha realm where all beings are in the form of the deity and all sounds are the sound of the deity's *mantra*. Generating a visualization of oneself as the deity, as in the generation stage of practice, one becomes a *vidyādhara* (knowledge holder) in the form of one's *yidam*. By this practice, one erodes the illusion of a fixed personal identity and learns how to close the door to future rebirth in a womb. As a *vidhyādhara*, one has the ability to travel to any Pure Land at will.

Padmasambhava's text describes several ways of "closing the entrance to the womb": (1) becoming a divine embodiment; (2) imagining your spiritual mentor with consort; (3) by the practice of the four blisses; (4) by the antidote of renunciation; (5) with the clear light; and (6) with the illusory body.[56] Due to habitual attachments to sexual desire, untrained sentient beings ordinarily and automatically gravitate to situations of sexual activity. One who will take rebirth as a female feels attracted to the male partner and one who will take rebirth as a male feels attracted to the female partner, and due to this sexual attraction enters the womb of one's future rebirth. However, if one is consciously able to turn away from the womb and visualize oneself in the form of a meditational deity in union with the deity's consort instead, it is possible to "block the entrance to the womb," meaning that one will not take rebirth in the ordinary way. Although rebirth may still occur, the practice sows the seeds for the achievement of *siddhis* (extraordinary accomplishments) both in the present and in future lifetimes, including the supreme *siddhi* of perfect enlightenment. The practices for closing the entrance to the womb are therefore one last opportunity for attaining realizations and final awakening.

Tibetan Interpretations of the Pure Land

The *Sukhāvatīvyūha Sūtra* is available in Tibetan translation, but it never achieved the prominence in Tibet that it did in East Asia. Prayers for rebirth in the Pure Land of Amitābha are recited daily in homes and monasteries throughout the Tibetan cultural region, but faith has never entirely supplanted effort in the quest for liberation. Prayers for rebirth in Dewachen, Amitābha's Pure Land, are recited in conjunction with the practice of *phowa* (*'pho ba*), the transference of consciousness at the moment of death. The meditative practice of *phowa* involves gathering the eighty-four thousand "winds" of the body into the central psychic channel (*uma*), and then directing the very subtle consciousness mounted on the very subtle wind through the Brahma aperture at the crown of the head and then on to a Pure Land where Buddhahood is ultimately attained.[57]

Rebirth in a Pure Land is acknowledged to be an accelerated and relatively simple alternative to the rigors of the *bodhisattva* path, but faith and practice are regarded as complementary, rather than oppositional. Faith (*śraddhā*) is a virtue, seen as a motivating force behind spiritual practice, but not as a goal in itself and not as a substitute for the hard work of mental cultivation. Devotional practices are highly valued in all Buddhist schools in Tibet, but scholarship and the arduous "graduated path to enlightenment" has generally been accorded pride of place. This valuation is reflected in the numerical and political dominance of the scholastic Gelug tradition. It is also reflected in the philosophical dominance of the dialectical method of the Prāsaṅgika Madhyamaka school.

Utilizing the *Bardo*

The concept of a *bardo* being who traverses an intermediary liminal stage between death and rebirth makes sense within a context that accepts *karma* and the recycling of consciousness as fundamental. Although Theravāda adherents deny the existence of such an interval and insist that rebirth occurs the moment after death ("arising-*citta* immediately follows falling-away-*citta*"), Peter Harvey finds evidence in the early texts to support the idea of an intermediate state.[58] In a passage from the *Saṃyutta Nikāya*, the Buddha refers to a time, fueled by craving, "when a being lays aside this body and is not arisen (*anuppanno*) in another body." Harvey shows that the time referred to here cannot be the period of gestation in the womb, because "arising" (*anuppanno*) can be distinguished from "becoming" (*bhava*), the condition for birth (*jāti*) in the twelve links of dependent arising (*pratītya-samutpāda*), which here refers to conception.[59] The Abhidharma asserts that both the mental and physical faculties (*indriya*) are present from the time of conception, and therefore conception is clearly the start of new life.[60] The *Saṃyutta Nikāya* passage leaves open the possibility of an interval between death and rebirth.

Even if the *bardo* being is impervious to physical harm, the relevant Tibetan texts make it clear that the body of the deceased should not be disturbed, since to disturb the body can disrupt the consciousness. Unless the dying person has developed excellent powers of concentration and compassion during the course of a lifetime, disturbances at the time of death are likely to distract the mind and can arouse fear or anger. Disturbing influences may affect the consciousness adversely and negatively influence the dying person's future rebirth. Although the person may be considered "deceased" and biologically dead by the medical staff and family members, in the Tibetan Buddhist view it is possible that the person's consciousness may continue to be active. A number of pertinent factors can affect a person's experiences during the dying process, at the time of death, in the *bardo* (should there be one), and in the next rebirth. These factors that can affect a person's transition from one life to the next include: (1) the circumstances leading to death; (2) the person's level of mental development; (3) the person's actions in the present and previous lifetimes; (4) the quality of the last moment of consciousness; and (5) the environment around the person during the transition. Let us consider these factors one by one.

First, the circumstances surrounding the death may be either peaceful or traumatic. Among the factors that determine this are whether the death is timely or untimely, whether the person is conscious or unconscious, and whether he or she is in pain or not. The most favorable circumstance for a peaceful transition is a death that results from natural causes and takes place in a pleasant environment. The least favorable circumstance for a peaceful transition is a sudden violent death that occurs in an atmosphere of fear, anger, or hatred.

Second, the person's level of mental development will determine what intellectual and contemplative resources the person brings to the experience of dying. The level of mental development can also determine, at least in part, whether the person is conscious or unconscious in the moments leading up to death, and whether the person is mindful at the moment of death and during the transition to the next rebirth, if there is one. The optimum circumstance, from a Buddhist point of view, exists for the practitioner who has gained mastery over the mind, eliminated all negative mental factors, cultivated all positive mental factors, and is able to die consciously. The worst circumstance exists when a person has no control over the mind, and is thus under the control of negative emotions, whether conscious or unconscious, and therefore cannot help but generate thoughts of anger and hatred during the process of dying.

From a Theravāda Buddhist perspective, the skilled practitioner described above will become an *arhat* without remainder (*nirupadhiśeṣanirvāṇa*), that is, will achieve liberation from rebirth and leave no aggregates behind. From a Mahāyāna perspective, the skilled practitioner will die peacefully and be able to concentrate on following the bright colored lights associated with the Buddhas, and as a result achieve either rebirth in a Pure Land or attain the perfect enlightenment of a Buddha. A Chinese Buddhist practitioner will achieve this through the practice of devotion to Amitābha Buddha; a Tibetan Buddhist practitioner will achieve this through the practice of *phowa*, *chö*, and various other tantric practices. All Buddhist traditions agree that a person who has no control over the mind will take rebirth at the mercy of *karma* and the delusions present in the mind. The *bardo* texts further state that beings who are unaware or frightened by their experiences will naturally gravitate, in accordance with their *karma*, to the dull lights associated with the six realms of rebirth.

Third, the person's actions in the present as well as in previous lifetimes will condition the experiences during the dying process and the *bardo*. A virtuous person will have accumulated the merit required to be reborn in a fortunate realm, whereas a nonvirtuous person will not have accumulated such merit, and will be reborn in an unfortunate realm. The strongest imprints on the mental continuum are said to ripen first and the imprints that are the most recent are likely to be the strongest.

Fourth, the quality of the last moment of consciousness is said to be a decisive factor in determining the quality of the next rebirth. For example, even if the circumstances of death are unfavorable, the person's past actions have been generally negative, and the mind is

untamed, there is still a possibility of generating a positive final moment of consciousness that could lead to a positive rebirth. Because
each moment of consciousness is conditioned by the moments that
have gone before it, the likelihood of an untrained, nonvirtuous person being able to generate a positive moment of consciousness, at this
critical juncture, is extremely unlikely, especially when the death occurs under unfavorable circumstances, such as violence. Still, according to the texts and commentaries, there is the possibility.

Finally, the environment surrounding a person facing death can
have a powerful influence. Even a skilled practitioner with good karma
who is dying a natural death under favorable conditions may experience an unwholesome moment of consciousness at the time of death,
due to some unexpected negative circumstance. If a person has developed perfect concentration, thoroughly eradicated all mental delusions,
and has developed all positive mental qualities, it is impossible for an
unwholesome consciousness to arise, for the person is either an *arhat*
or a Buddha and therefore not subject to rebirth, or a *bodhisattva* and
therefore not subject to uncontrolled rebirth. A person who has not
attained these qualities, however, is vulnerable to outside influences,
and so it is possible that an unwholesome consciousness may arise.
Even a highly skilled practitioner can conceivably be affected by anger, hatred, or desire and may, as a result, generate an unfavorable
last moment of consciousness. Similarly, a person who has negative
karma and an uncontrolled, nonvirtuous mind is vulnerable to outside
influences and may generate a wholesome last moment of consciousness. For example, such a person could conceivably be affected by a
calm, loving, and compassionate immediate environment that results
in the generation of a positive state of mind at the moment of death.

For this reason, Buddhists are concerned with creating a peaceful, loving environment for the dying. A teacher or spiritual friend
may be invited to advise the dying person in accordance with Buddha's
teachings, and especially to remind the person that death and dissolution are inevitable for all living beings. Chinese and Tibetan Buddhists may place images of enlightenment, such as Buddhas and
bodhisattvas, within the dying person's range of vision. Family and
friends who believe in the efficacy of merit will make offerings to
monasteries and the Saṅgha, donate charity to the needy, chant *sūtras*
or prayers or the Buddha's name, and dedicate the merits of these
practices to the dying or just deceased person. All these efforts are
aimed at creating a favorable environment, accumulating positive *karma*,
and nurturing a positive state of mind to ensure a favorable transition
from this life to the next. Even those who are not convinced about the

existence of future lives, the efficacy of merit, the existence of the *bardo*, or the possibility of attaining higher rebirth and enlightenment generally feel that it is worthwhile to observe these traditions, just in case there may be some benefit.

The result of these beliefs and practices is fulfilling, both personally and socially. For example, providing a serene environment in which the trajectory of death can occur brings a sense of peace and well-being not only to the dying person, but to the family and friends as well. To conduct one's life in accordance with Buddhist guidelines (i.e., to engage in wholesome actions and avoid unwholesome ones, and cultivate mental discipline, concentration, and compassion) helps to allay everyone's fears about a person's future after death and can put the mind in a positive frame at the moment of death. To engage in positive actions on behalf of the deceased, such as the practice of generosity, recitation of *sūtras*, and other meritorious actions, is psychologically beneficial for survivors, and helps to alleviate grief, and the sense of loss, or remorse. In this way, Buddhist beliefs and rituals are of practical benefit for both the dying person and the family. As an added benefit, if there is a *bardo*, the deceased is in a position to direct the transition with maximum skill and benefit. And, if there is a future life, the deceased is more assured of a favorable one. Therefore, setting aside questions about its ontological status, the *bardo* concept may prove valuable in facilitating a positive experience of dying.

Chapter 8

The Ethical Urgency
of Death

Philosophical perspectives and popular beliefs about death and the nature of what occurs after death set the stage for an exploration of bioethical issues from Buddhist points of view. This exploration requires, first, an examination of traditional textual sources to see what they say about specific bioethical questions and, second, reflection on the application of Buddhist ethical ideals to current social and technological realities. Although Buddhist ethical theory is clear on certain issues, such as abortion, other issues such as an examination of the ethics of suicide and assisted suicide, organ transplantation, and stem cell research are less clear-cut. This reveals the complexity of biomedical ethics throughout and the variety of Buddhist perspectives both in the texts and in different Buddhist cultures. These cultures developed independently in far-flung regions of Asia among people who valued contemplation more than technology. In the absence of a central bureaucracy for vetting ideas, it was left to individual monks and monasteries to formulate Buddhist responses to ethical dilemmas. Today, as Buddhist ideas spread around the world, people from many different backgrounds are formulating new applications of Buddhist principles to address issues of common human concern.

Many of the ethical dilemmas that arise as a result of advanced medical technologies are not specifically addressed in the ancient Buddhist texts, simply because these technologies did not exist when those texts were written. Buddha Śākyamuni did not speak about genetic engineering or assisted reproduction, so any exploration of these dilemmas from a Buddhist perspective requires us to study them first within the context of traditional Buddhist ethical theory as a whole and then to extrapolate from there. The Buddhist codes of ethics must be interpreted in view of such changes. In the absence of categorical imperatives and higher sources of authority, a critical analysis of these topics forces us to move beyond the received moral guidelines and to think in new, sometimes uncomfortable directions. The exercise is an essential and timely one, since new technologies are likely to continue appearing that will require Buddhists to stretch their thinking even further.

Building the Framework: The Basis of Traditional Buddhist Ethics

The Buddha taught an ethic of personal responsibility in which individuals are accountable for their actions as well as the results of their actions, the law of cause and effect. The precepts are guidelines for ethical conduct, rather than moral absolutes. Ethics are situational and relational, but there is a baseline for ordinary decision making and a moral consistency that underlies the various formulations of ethical precepts. Buddhists generally regard ethical (virtuous) actions as having an impact in three ways: they reduce the negative tendencies of the mind; they foster positive tendencies conducive to future happiness and liberation (nirvāṇa); and they contribute to the harmonious functioning of society. Even though actions and attitudes are conditioned by circumstances and by predispositions resulting from actions created in the past, individuals are theoretically free to choose either wholesome actions that result in happiness or unwholesome actions that result in unhappiness. Maximizing the benefits of positive actions and mitigating the deleterious effects of negative actions are primary aims of Buddhist spiritual practice and Buddhist ethics, and these practical concerns are more important than theoretical concerns.

Among the wide range of contemporary approaches to decision making among Buddhists, the common denominator is the principle of cause and effect. According to this principle, karma ripens inexorably and there is no way to escape the results of one's deeds. No effect ripens without a cause, and, given suitable conditions, there is no cause that does not produce consequences. The effects of one's actions cannot ripen on another person, and another person's actions cannot ripen on you. Virtuous action can mitigate the intensity of the effects, but cannot cancel them out altogether. This general explication of the workings of cause and effect is common to all Buddhists traditions.

Four specific criteria determine when an action is complete and will therefore result in the fullest possible consequences: object, intention, action, and completion of the action. First, one must ascertain the object of the action, for example, a frog. Second, one must generate the intention to commit the action, for example, the intention to kill the frog. Third, one must carry through with the action; in this case, one must kill the frog. Fourth, one must feel satisfied that the action is complete; in this case, one must ascertain and experience satisfaction that the frog is dead. When all four criteria are present, the action is considered complete and the doer of the action accrues the full consequences of the action. If any of the four criteria are absent, the consequences of the action are mitigated to some degree. For example, if one mistakes a rock for a frog, the action of killing a frog is not committed, even if the other criteria are present. If a frog is killed unintentionally, the second criteria is absent, even if the other three are present. If the action is not carried through to completion, the third criteria is not fulfilled. If there is no feeling of satisfaction at having killed the frog, even when the first three criteria are present, the action is not complete. In all these cases of mitigating circumstances, the action is considered incomplete and the consequences of the action are correspondingly less severe.

Buddhist ethics is couched in a nontheistic metaphysics, with no creator God who judges, rewards, or punishes. Buddhas (fully awakened beings), *bodhisattvas* (aspirants on the path to Buddhahood), and *arhats* (liberated beings) do not control or sit in judgment of others. Instead, individuals are free and responsible to choose their actions (*karma*) of body, speech, and mind, which are subject to the impersonal law of cause and effect. Tangled within the complex web of actions and the results of actions created by infinite beings throughout the universe, individuals have the potential to avoid the unskillful actions that lead to suffering, to engage in the skillful actions that lead to happiness, and to ultimately free themselves from the cycle of rebirth.

There are two categories of misdeeds in Buddhist ethical thinking, natural and formulated. The first type, natural misdeeds (Tibetan: *rang bzhin gyi kha na ma tho ba*), refers to conduct that is regarded as nonvirtuous by people, lay or ordained, regardless of where or when they live, for example, killing a human being, stealing the property of another, and rape. The second type, formulated misdeeds (Tibetan: *bcas pa'i kha na ma tho ba*), refers to faults that arise from transgressing precepts or principles that one has agreed to observe. Formulated misdeeds vary according to time, place, and circumstance. In the Buddhist traditions, laypeople, novices, and fully ordained monastics abide by various formulations of precepts. These voluntary rules of training serve as behavioral guidelines for assessing what constitutes a wholesome or unwholesome action of body, speech, or mind. Some of these formulations of precepts are temporary observances, whereas others are lifelong commitments. The five precepts for laypeople serve as a baseline of Buddhist ethics: to refrain from taking life, stealing, sexual misconduct, false speech, and intoxicants. Although taking intoxicants is considered the least serious of the five precepts, intoxicants cloud the mind and thus make one more prone to commit other infractions. Tibetans tell the story of a handsome young monk who, while walking along a forest path, was confronted by a woman leading a goat and holding a vessel of wine. The woman threatened to commit suicide unless the monk either drank the wine, killed the goat, or slept with her, all three of which were breaches of his monastic precepts. Assuming that the wine was the least serious option, he drank it and wound up committing all three transgressions.

The ethical framework for distinguishing wholesome and unwholesome actions is broadly defined by the injunctions of the Noble Eightfold Path: right view, right intention, right speech, right action, right livelihood, right effort, right mindfulness, and right concentration. Ethical injunctions are also codified in the ten virtuous actions, the Prātimokṣa precepts, and similar formulations. Broadly speaking, Buddhist ethics encompasses all wholesome actions and good qualities, including faith, mindfulness, energy, and wisdom. In another formulation, pure moral discipline involves morality (śīla), restraint of the senses (indriya-saṃvara), mindfulness (sati-sampajañña), and contentment (santuṭṭhi). Ultimately, the value of Buddhist ethics is practical: to forestall acts of violence, deceit, aggression, negativity, impropriety, and regret. Advocating a middle path between asceticism and self-indulgence, repression and debauchery, Buddhist moral discipline invests the individual with responsibility for developing the wisdom to determine the appropriate action in a particular context.

The Prātimokṣa texts also include more specific behavioral guidelines. These include five precepts for male and laypeople (upāsaka or upāsikā), ten precepts for novice monks and nuns (śrāmaṇera or śrāmaṇerikā), over two hundred precepts for fully ordained monks (bhikṣu), and over three hundred for fully ordained nuns (bhikṣuṇī). An additional category is the twenty-four-hour lay precepts (upavāsaka). The five precepts of a Buddhist layperson are to refrain from taking life, taking what is not given, telling lies, sexual misconduct, and intoxicants. The ten precepts of a novice monk or nun are to refrain from taking life, taking what is not given, telling lies, sexual activity of any sort, intoxicants, singing and dancing, ornaments and cosmetics, high or luxurious seats and beds, handling gold and silver, and taking untimely food. The additional precepts of a fully ordained monk or nun seem intended to protect the monastic order (Saṅgha) from harm, to avoid criticism from the lay community, and to ensure the harmonious functioning and continuation of the order. Bi-monthly gatherings with a confession of faults and recitation of precepts help to maintain high standards of conduct and ethical integrity. The Prātimokṣa precepts provide a groundwork for moral behavior that helps create harmonious communities and eventually leads to individual liberation.

The Mahāyāna emphasis on *bodhicitta* and emptiness results in some elaborations in ethical thinking. The concepts of *bodhicitta* (the altruistic intention to achieve perfect awakening in order to free all sentient beings from suffering) and *śūnyatā* (the lack of true existence of all phenomena) give the *bodhisattva* an exponentially more complex frame of reference for making ethical decisions. According to this line of thinking, there may be occasions when the *bodhisattva* intention to liberate all beings from suffering may be thought to supersede the Prātimokṣa precepts that ordinarily guide Buddhist ethical decision making. In such cases, a *bodhisattva* may be willing to commit an infraction of the lay or monastic precepts in order to benefit living beings or alleviate their suffering, even though the *bodhisattva* accumulates unwholesome *karma* as a result of doing so. To illustrate, a person with perfect compassion might be willing to risk or to suffer the consequences of an action of killing or stealing—even the torments of hell for a very long time—to relieve the sufferings of a specific sentient being. For example, a *bodhisattva* theoretically may be willing to risk a hellish rebirth by taking the life of a puppy who is suffering from distemper. The risks of this line of reasoning are not hard to see, since a person could try to justify virtually any nonvirtuous action by claiming a higher intention. But theoretically at least, the parameters of such a decision are clear; Mahāyāna ethics are used to justify an unwholesome action only if the motivation is purely to benefit others and prevent their suffering. Further, the doer of the action must be fully aware of the likely consequences of the action and have the courage and compassion to accept those consequences. Typically, it is only *bodhisattvas* who have such a high degree of courage, wisdom, and compassion.

Among Tibetan Buddhists, the Prātimokṣa precepts are generally viewed as the foundation of ethics and there is little support for the idea of assisted suicide. In most situations, although one is free to choose, suicide and assisted suicide are viewed as misguided courses of action. At the same time, Tibetan Buddhists maintain the *bodhisattva* ideal and regard *bodhisattvas* as exceptional beings who consistently value the welfare of other beings more than their own. Two conflicting views of *bodhisattva* ethics may emerge. On one hand, *bodhisattvas* are motivated by the purest possible intention, *bodhicitta*, and therefore may decide to commit a nonvirtuous action or breach of the precepts in order to spare a particular sentient being from harm. On the other hand, motivated by the pure *bodhicitta* intention to liberate all beings, one may choose to avoid all misdeeds, expiate all nonvirtuous *karma* as quickly as possible, and achieve perfect enlightenment without delay, since a Buddha is most capable of effecting the highest benefit of all beings.

The principle of cause and effect is often portrayed as an inexorable law, such that one inevitably experiences the results of one's actions. In the Tibetan tradition, however, there is a time-honored method of expiating or mitigating the effects of one's actions by applying the Four Opponent Powers. One sets the stage for this practice by visualizing a host of Buddhas and *bodhisattvas* in the space before one. In the presence of this illustrious pantheon, one acknowledges one's misdeed, then generates sincere feelings of regret and remorse for having committed the action, then makes a strong resolution not to repeat the misdeed, and finally, engages in some form of Dharma practice to offset the negative effects of the action. This virtuous activity may take the form of meditation, an act of generosity, the recitation of texts or *mantras*, or some similar type of practice. Whether the karmic effects of the misdeed are totally eradicated or are simply mitigated in some way is unclear and may depend on the seriousness of the offense and the sincerity of one's remorse. The straightforward confession of faults underscores personal accountability; remorse and the determination not to repeat the action encourage a transformation in behavior, and the practice of some virtuous activity as an antidote helps eliminates feelings of guilt.

Among Buddhists, it is believed that a person who is totally enlightened will naturally behave in an ethical way. In some traditions, it is even believed that, by virtue of being enlightened, a person acts spontaneously for the highest good, sometimes transgressing the conventional ethical constraints that apply to ordinary beings still on the path. An example from the tantric tradition is the realized Indian *yogi* Tilopa who popped live fish into his mouth and swallowed them whole. When castigated for such cruel behavior, Tilopa displayed his yogic attainments by regurgitating the fish alive, thus demonstrating that he was beyond conventional ethical strictures. The point of the story is that, under certain circumstances, apparent transgressions may be the enlightened activity of a Buddha, *bodhisattva*, or other realized being. Since it is difficult to know for sure who is a realized being and who is not, it may be wise to withhold moral judgment about the actions of others. On the other hand, according to conventional ethics, killing a sentient being is unambiguously nonvirtuous, so for ordinary (unenlightened) beings, the wisest course may be to simply follow the precepts.

The Buddhist focus on taking life is not simply a mandate. Taking life is undesirable because it causes suffering. Every living being, even the smallest ant, cherishes its own life and wants to avoid dying. To deprive a sentient being of its life not only causes suffering, but also interrupts that being's life cycle and its migration within cyclic existence, which is an unwarranted imposition of one being's wishes upon another. Further, taking life is a grievously unwholesome action that results in unfortunate consequences for the one who kills. The combination of these factors leads Buddhists to refrain from taking the life of any sentient being, no matter how small. Based on the injunction to refrain from taking life and the premise that life begins at conception, Buddhists typically avoid abortion, euthanasia, suicide, or any other action that involves intentionally killing a sentient being, whether human, animal, or insect.

The various Buddhist schools concur that nothing is more dear to a sentient being than its own life. For this reason, Buddhists attempt to live in ways that protect living creatures and their habitats. In the Buddhist context, possessing consciousness is the distinguishing characteristic of a sentient being. Animals, fish, and insects are sentient beings, but plant life is not, though plants may have sentient beings closely associated with them. To respect and protect life, even that of the smallest creature, is thought to create the causes for long life, good health, and a pleasant living environment in this and future lives. Saving the lives of animals by purchasing them from the butcher or the fishmonger is a time-honored custom among Buddhists, especially in China, Tibet, and other Mahāyāna countries. Ceremonies for "liberating life" have become especially popular in Taiwan in recently years, with special concern for tortoises. Buddhists in China, Korea, and Vietnam express their concern for animals by maintaining a vegetarian (often vegan) diet as a natural expression of nonviolence and a logical extension of the precept against taking life. The strong commitment to preserving life has remained unchanged over centuries of Buddhist historical development and has led Buddhists to maintain their nonviolent ideals even in the face of aggression, as shown by events in Burma, Thailand, Tibet, and elsewhere in the last century.

Despite their philosophical and cultural differences, all Buddhists strive to maintain the nonviolent ideal of refraining from harm.

A core principle for both Buddhist monastics and laity is to refrain from taking life. The reasoning behind this injunction is that nothing is as dear to a living being as its own life and to deprive a being of its life is a source of great suffering, both for the being who is killed and for the killer, due to the unfortunate consequences of killing. The behavior of animals on their way to the slaughterhouse and insects about to be squashed is ample evidence that living beings cherish their lives and do not wish to be harmed or killed. The injunction against taking life is therefore rooted in compassion for the sufferings of living beings—not only for the victim who suffers being killed, but for the perpetrator who must suffer the consequences of an act of killing, such as a rebirth in a hellish realm (naraka). The immediate result is rebirth in a lower realm; the result consistent with the cause is that later, having achieved a human rebirth, one will have a short life with many illnesses and a predilection for killing; the environmental result is that later, in a human life, food and medicines will not be nutritious or effective.[1] Buddhist texts and teachers invoke the principle of non-harm (ahiṃsa), to refrain from harming any sentient life, and the principle of benefiting sentient beings, to act with compassion to relieve the suffering of all living creatures. Both on the grounds of non-harm and compassion, Buddhists strive to avoid taking the life of any sentient being.

The most serious instance of taking life is to take the life of a human being. A being who has achieved a perfect human rebirth is capable of understanding the principle of cause and effect, of distinguishing wholesome from unwholesome deeds, and of making intelligent decisions. The intense sufferings of the hell beings, the intense pleasures of the gods, and the deep stupidity of animals prevent these creatures from being able to distinguish between ethical and unethical modes of conduct. As a result, the beings in these states of rebirth continue to revolve through countless rebirths with little chance of extricating themselves. Human beings, because of their intelligence and their capacity for logical reasoning, have the capacity to liberate themselves from the wheel of rebirth, and therefore are regarded as the most fortunate of sentient life forms.

Due to the advantages of a human existence, human beings play a central role in Buddhist soteriology, but it would not be justified to label Buddhism anthropocentric, since all living beings are cherished and equally valued. In the Buddhist texts there is ample evidence of the value placed on animal life. For example, the precepts in the Vinaya (the monastic codes of discipline) prohibit fully ordained monastics from intentionally taking the life of a creature belonging to the animal kingdom, pouring water containing living creatures on grass, clay, or earth (or having someone else do so), cutting down large trees (because they may be the habitat of living creatures), and knowingly using water that contains living creatures. Monastics are required to strain their drinking water to avoid taking the lives of even the smallest creature; one of their requisites is a water strainer for this purpose. All human beings have experienced rebirth as an animal innumerable times and it is therefore easy to imagine the sufferings that animals undergo and to generate compassion for them. Even so, a human existence is most highly prized, because in the Buddhist ethical framework intelligent human beings are most qualified to act as moral agents. For this reason, to take the life of a human being is the most serious of nonvirtues and to refrain from taking human life is the cardinal moral principle.

Along with the firm commitment to preserving life among Buddhists, there is strong agreement that individuals are responsible for their own actions and decisions. Because individuals themselves experience the results of their actions, they have both the freedom and the responsibility to determine the appropriateness of those actions. Although Buddhist texts do not use the language of rights and prerogatives, an analysis of the theory of *karma* makes it clear that human beings act as a moral agents and are responsible for their own decisions. There is a sense that moral behavior can be taught and nurtured, and families and monasteries serve precisely that purpose. The conditions of one's life situation may be more or less favorable, but ultimately each person determines his or her own future direction. Although families and monasteries have conventions and rules that members are expected to follow, morality is not legislated by any higher authority. For this reason, many of the arguments advanced by contemporary ethicists concerning the permissibility of actions do not find exact parallels within the Buddhist context. For example, the concept of "playing God" assumes the existence of a higher power whose authority would be challenged by human beings who performed actions of a similar order, but such a being does not figure into Buddhist discussions of ethical decision making. Instead, decisions are weighed according to the moral guidelines set forth by the Buddha, consistent with the law of cause and effect.

A cross-cultural analysis of bioethics first requires a cross-cultural analysis of the nature of death and the afterlife. The belief that death is a final end or a passageway to paradise, for example, sets the stage for a different set of responses to bioethical issues than does a view of death based on multiple lifetimes and rebirths. For instance, if human beings' actions have no effect beyond this one lifetime, then there may be no compelling reason to restrain one's desires and antipathies. In the absence of rewards or punishments in the afterlife, public legislation and the penal system may serve the function of moral arbitrator in preventing or penalizing socially destructive words and deeds. From a Buddhist perspective, the law of cause and effect may be a more just and cost-effective regulator of moral conduct than legal structures, in that the consequences of an individual's actions extend beyond death.

Within a Buddhist moral framework, individuals are taught to internalize the parameters of acceptable behavior and make their own decisions accordingly, recognizing that the consequences of actions rebound on themselves. Although there is no way to document it conclusively, the law of cause and effect is thought to operate over many lifetimes, but it does not play out in a strictly linear or chronological way. Good things may happen to bad people and bad things may happen to good people, because the seeds of past actions do not necessarily ripen sequentially. Good fortune in this lifetime is not necessarily the consequence of virtuous actions in the immediate past lifetime, but may have been created many lifetimes ago. Similarly, wholesome and unwholesome actions created in the present may come to fruition in this lifetime *or* they may be experienced in some future life. In other words, there is no way to precisely predict the timing or circumstances in which the consequence of a specific action will ripen. Understanding the workings of cause and effect in this way, Buddhists generally do not lapse into despair in the face of hardships even in circumstances of pain, poverty, or oppression. The unaccountable cheerfulness of H. H. Dalai Lama despite the cultural genocide and injustices of communist rule in Tibet is an example of applying these principles to explain and cope with the difficulties of life.

From a traditional Buddhist standpoint, it is therefore wise to avoid every unskillful action, no matter how small, especially the action of taking life. The problems that one experiences at present are the result of actions taken in the past, just as unskillful actions created in this lifetime will result in problems in the future. To commit suicide as a means of alleviating mental or physical suffering is misguided, because the suffering in the next existence may be even greater, especially as a result of committing suicide. One may feel justified in taking one's own life or even that of another in order to avoid suffering now, but unfortunately such an action will only compound one's future misery. Suicide is by no means an easy way out and killing even in self-defense is not recommended. Ultimately, the only way to avoid suffering is to avoid being born, and to become free from rebirth, one must be exceedingly careful about every action.

Cross-denominational Buddhist Attitudes toward Taking Life

Buddhist attitudes on issues of life and death are embedded in a metaphysics of *karma* and rebirth, but each Buddhist tradition is also simultaneously situated in a unique cultural narrative. The Buddhist traditions share many theoretical assumptions and ethical principles in common, but each operates within a unique and continually evolving hermeneutical context. The twenty-first-century convergence of Buddhism and contemporary cultures that is occurring today in Paris, Bangkok, San Francisco, and other locations around the world is but the most recent phase of an ongoing process of interpretation, adaptation, and evolution that began soon after the Buddha's own lifetime. While Buddhists today may invoke early textual traditions and codes of behavior as guideposts for contemporary reflection and action, the conversation about how the Buddhist teachings apply to current lifestyles and different cultural contexts is just beginning. For example, Buddhists in Sri Lanka, Japan, and the United States may approach the topic of suicide from very different angles, based on their social, cultural, and psychological backgrounds. This diversity of attitudes and experiences will require patient understanding, but will make for a very rich dialogue.

Buddhists have just begun to discuss and to articulate an acceptable range of ethical options in response to new ethical complexities. As medical technologies have become more sophisticated, the dying process has become longer and more complicated than in earlier times. In a very short time, decisions about amniocentesis, artificial insemination, feeding tubes, ventilators, and advance health care directives have entered the public consciousness and presented individuals, families, and hospitals around the world with new and increasingly complex decisions. The time lag between East and West has become truncated, and as new technologies become readily available in Asia or are developed there, people are beginning to face some of the same ethical dilemmas that face people in North America and Europe. As the human life span increases, in more developed countries at least, terminally ill patients and their families are confronted with decisions about whether or not to seek medical means of prolonging life, and whether and when to terminate artificial life support once it is begun. An increasing number of terminally ill patients are seeking hospice care, while others are deciding they do not wish to outlive their usefulness.

Analyzing contemporary attitudes toward suicide and assisted suicide is valuable, because the arguments raised in relation to these issues may help us think about other bioethical questions. For example, according to one stream of Buddhist opinion on the question of suicide and assisted suicide, the state of the dying person's consciousness at the moment of death is more significant than the action of suicide itself. If the intention is pure (say, to save one's family the high cost of nursing care), the action of suicide may have no ill effects, because it is the pure intention that will become implanted in one's mental continuum and will bear fruit in the future. One has the right to make life and death decisions, they argue, because one is accountable for one's own actions and will ultimately experience the results of one's actions.

According to another stream of opinion, suicide and assisted suicide are never advisable. If one decides on suicide or assisted suicide in an attempt to escape suffering, the decision is considered unwise for several reasons. First, one cannot escape the unpleasant consequences of one's previous actions so easily. If the unpleasant consequences of one's actions are not either experienced or purified in some way, one will experience them at some future time. Second, one accrues the negative karma of killing oneself, a seriously nonvirtuous action that will result in even greater suffering in the future. Third, by assisting someone to commit suicide, another person (usually a physician or caregiver) also commits an action of killing and will experience the unpleasant consequences. Fourth, the state of mind of a terminal patient who decides to take her/his own life may be fuzzy or distorted due to any number of factors, including medications and depression, so the decision may not be clearly thought through. There is one possible exception: If the consciousness of both parties is clear and free of any distortion, and their intentions are absolutely pure (for example, they are *bodhisattvas*), it is possible that the outcome will be positive, or at least not negative. However, for the ordinary person the outcome will be miserable.

Evolving a Buddhist Bioethics

Among Buddhists, the ideologies of individual concern and social concern merge in the practice of the *bodhisattva* ideal, found in the Pāli canon and further emphasized in Mahāyāna texts. This ethical ideal, which seeks the welfare of both self and others, culminates in the achievement of human perfection known as awakening or enlightenment. Buddhist philosophical systems vary in theory and tone, but they share similar metaphysical foundations that date from the Buddha's time, or even before, and a shared body of ethical principles premised on non-harm. These are the fundamental assumptions and ethical principles that Buddhists of the various traditions bring to their assessments of bioethical issues, and Buddhists are just beginning to discuss how these assumptions and principles can be used to analyze the difficult questions raised by new technologies. Since these technologies are being developed on the basis of a very different set of assumptions and values, the task is extremely challenging.

In the Pāli texts, it is clear that the Buddha did not sanction suicide. The suicides described in the early Buddhist texts were committed by individuals due to feelings of disgust toward the human body, misunderstandings about the theory of no-self, frustrations about their spiritual progress, or intense pain accompanying a serious illness. For example, the Vinaya relates the story about certain monks who became so filled with loathing while meditating on the unpleasant nature of the body that they took their own lives. When the Buddha discovered this, he condemned suicide in no uncertain terms and recommended that his disciples practice mindfulness of breathing instead.

To commit suicide is not classified as a *pārājika* in the Vinaya, because the precepts are described as based on the wrongdoings of specific monks and nuns, and in the case of a suicide there is no surviving individual to censure. However, there are passages in the Vinaya that censure monks for aiding, abetting, or encouraging suicide. This proscription came about after a group of monks encouraged certain laypeople to commit suicide, saying that they would enjoy the fruits of their good *karma* sooner that way. The actions of aiding, abetting, or encouraging suicide are censored as equivalent to taking the life of a human being and are punishable by expulsion from the monastic order. This confirms that taking one's own life is equivalent to taking another human being's life and equally censurable.

The third *pārājika* (defeat or root downfall) for a fully ordained nun or monk is to take the life of a human being and is grounds for expulsion from the monastic order. This precept not only proscribes the action of killing a human being, but also the actions of arranging to have someone killed, and assisting or encouraging someone to kill. In the *Bhikṣuṇī Pratimokṣa Sūtra* of the Tibetan Mūlasarvāstivādin school, the precept explicitly states:

> If a *bhikṣuṇī* intentionally takes the life of a human being or
> a fetus with her own hands, gives a weapon to someone,
> incites someone to take up a weapon, urges death, or praises

death, saying, "Why live such a foul, dreadful, nonvirtuous
life? It would be easier to die than to live such a life," then
at the time it is done, that *bhikṣuṇī* commits a *pārājika* and
is expelled from the order.[2]

Suicide is proscribed because it takes the life of a human being, even
when it is carried out in ignorance of the negative karmic consequences.
Because a human rebirth is necessary for progress on the path to liberation, and is so rare and difficult to attain, suicide is contrary to the
benefit of living beings and their achievement of liberation. Suicide
may end suffering in this life, but it ignores the unpleasant long-term
consequences of the action that extend to future rebirths. Considerable
merit is required to acquire higher states of rebirth, and it is tragic to
waste such a fortunate opportunity. Moreover, even though one may
contemplate suicide as a remedy for the sufferings of this life, it is
possible that one will be reborn in a situation even more miserable
than the one at hand. Buddhists therefore view suicide as both misguided and futile.

Buddhist ethical decision making on end-of-life issues is therefore thoroughly grounded in the proscription against taking the life
of sentient beings, especially the life of human beings. This prohibition is based on two premises: first, sentient beings suffer when they
are deprived of their lives, and second, sentient beings possess the
rare potential to achieve liberation and the actualization of this potential is disrupted by an untimely death. The first premise is
grounded on compassion for the sufferings of sentient beings; the
second is grounded on the idea that, among sentient beings, human
beings enjoy a special status and the potential to liberate themselves
and others from suffering once and for all. While these principles
form the basis for a Buddhist theoretical analysis of bioethical decision making, mitigating circumstances and the intentions that motivate actions are also taken into account. Certain Chinese Mahāyāna
texts mention suicides motivated by altruism and devotion, but for
ordinary beings suicide is classified as a seriously nonvirtuous action that is to be avoided.

Given this background, it is surprising to find several passages
in the early scriptures in which the Buddha apparently respected a
terminally ill monk's choice to die. In the Pāli canon we find the cases
of three monks—Vakkali, Godhika, and Channa—who, in seeking release from the extreme suffering of acute illness, put an end to their
lives with knives.[3] The Buddha apparently exonerated these suicides
and posthumously declared the monks to be *arhats*. In another similar

passage, the monk Assaji became so debilitated that he was no longer able to control the pain through the practice of *samādhi*, and so he cut his own throat. After his death, again, the Buddha confirmed that Assaji had attained the state of an *arhat*. These passages describe the suicides of three monks who were *arhats* and suffering from extremely painful illnesses. In the absence of pain medications such as those available today, it appears that the Buddha exonerated or at least failed to condemn acts of suicide committed by monks who were in acute pain from a terminal illness and who either had achieved the fruit of the path or were on the brink of achieving it. Although the Buddha did not encourage suicide, he apparently did not prevent it either, at least in these cases of terminal illness with excruciating pain.

In all of these cases, the monks received teachings on impermanence and suffering prior to their deaths. Presumably these teachings were given to help them maintain their practice of mindfulness, which is crucial at the moment of death to prevent one from grasping at another existence. The fact that these monks became *arhats*, a non-regressive state of liberation from suffering and rebirth, indicates that they did not accumulate negative karma by committing suicide. Under ordinary circumstances, practitioners are obliged to preserve their lives, in order to benefit themselves and others; actions inevitably give rise to consequences and the unwholesome action of killing would lead to an unfortunate rebirth. Therefore, these monks must have attained the state of an *arhat* either sometime prior to committing suicide or at the very moment of their death; if they had not already achieved liberation from *saṃsāra*, the action of committing suicide would have entailed further rebirth.

Citing the *Pāyāsi Sutta*, Martin G. Wiltshire contends that the body is merely the receptacle of the consciousness. Its purpose is "to allow for one's own spiritual development and to assist others," but "should the body reach that condition or point at which it can no longer perform these functions—as in the case of an incurable malady or illness—then death becomes little more than de jure confirmation of a de facto situation." Before each of the cases of suicide cited above, the Buddha asks whether the monk has any anxiety or ethical transgressions to confess, since, in Wiltshire's words, "to die with a bad conscience is kammically lethal." According to this text, the Buddha pronounced these three monks "blameless (*anupavājja*)," consonant with their achievement of liberation. Wiltshire concludes that a properly motivated person who has realized impermanence and no-self can be condoned for relinquishing a spent body through suicide. This view is not shared by most Buddhists, however.

The Ethics of Self-Immolation

One of the strongest challenges to traditional Buddhist ethics is the incidence of self-immolation among Buddhists in China and Vietnam. Despite the Buddha's injunctions against suicide, there are cases of Buddhists who have set their bodies afire as an act of generosity, renunciation, devotion, or political protest. The practice of self-immolation did not gain currency in India, but references to the practice can be found in the Mahāyāna texts *Saddharmapuṇḍarīka Sūtra* and *Mahāprajñāpāramitā-śāstra*, and in two apocryphal texts that became extremely influential in China, the *Fanwangjing* and the *Shoulangyanjing*.[4] Despite the fact that taking life and advocating suicide are both clearly proscribed in the Vinaya texts, these Mahāyāna texts extol the virtues of offering one's body to the Buddhas, often by burning. The *bodhisattva* Bhaiṣajyarāja's autocremation in the *Saddharmapuṇḍarīka Sūtra* is unequivocally portrayed as a virtuous act. Yet despite the Indian origins of such texts as the *Saddharmapuṇḍarika-sūtra*, Chinese pilgrims reported that self-immolation and self-mutilation were not practiced in India as they were in China.[5] In his pioneering study, Jan Yün-hua mentions that there are many documented incidents of self-immolation by eminent nuns and monks that occurred in Chinese Buddhist history. It is Jan's opinion that the incidents of physical self-sacrifice that appear in the texts were meant as hyperbole, but were taken literally by the Chinese. Sporadic incidents of the practice have been reported up to recent times.

The first documented self-immolation in China may have occurred as early as the fourth century, when the monk Fayu first ate incense and then burnt himself to death as an offering to the Buddha while chanting a section of the *Saddharmapuṇḍarīka Sūtra*.[6] Jan notes two precursors of this practice in China: moxibustion and ritual autocremation in supplication for rain.[7] Although the practice diametrically contradicts the Buddha's exhortation to abandon extreme asceticism, the sixteenth precept of the apocryphal *Fanwangjing* states explicitly that a *bodhisattva* should teach ascetic practices such as setting fire to a finger, arm, or the whole body or offering one's limbs and flesh to wild animals and hungry ghosts as an act of renunciation.[8]

Early Chinese Buddhist accounts of self-immolations testify that the practice was often highly valued. The *Biquini zhuan* (*Lives of the Nuns*) gives several examples. On a full moon night in 463:

> Tao-tsung [Daozong], as an offering to the Buddha, purified herself in a fire fed by oil. Even though she was en-

gulfed by flames up to her forehead, and her eyes and ears were nearly consumed, her chanting of the scriptures did not falter. Monastics and householders sighed in wonder; the demonic and upright were alike startled. When the country heard this news, everyone aspired to attain enlightenment. The appointed court scholar of Sung [Song], Liu Ch'iu [Liuqiu] (438–495), especially revered her and composed a Buddhist-style poetic verse to praise her.[9]

Although these incidents inspired awe, they also caused consternation and sadness. A contemplative nun named Tanjian, who was renowned for her virtue, often collected firewood, "saying that she was going to carry out a meritorious act," then one day in 494:

> . . . [S]he mounted this pile of firewood and kindled a fire, immolating herself, thereby abandoning her body of birth and death as an offering to the Three Treasures. When the people in the neighboring village saw the fire, they raced to rescue her, but, when they arrived, T'an-chien [Tanjian] had already died. Religious and laity alike lamented, their cries reverberating through the mountains and valleys.[10]

Another nun from the same convent, Jinggui, burned her body at the same time:

> She was pure in conduct, broadly versed in both the scriptures and the monastic rules, and well accomplished in all the meditative secrets of the three types of Buddhist paths [*śrāvaka*, *pratyekabuddha*, and *bodhisattva*]. . . . Religious and laity, all grieving and weeping, collected her relics and buried them in a tomb.[11]

The psychology that motivated these immolations and the impact created in Tang Chinese society by the immolations of such highly accomplished and respected practitioners, can only be imagined.

Confucian society strongly condemned self-destruction and self-mutilation, but to die for one's principles was highly respected. During a visit to China in 1982, I heard many stories of nuns who committed suicide to avoid rape either by troops or marauders during the chaos of the 1940s and the Cultural Revolution. In Chinese societies, it is generally presumed that the "spirit" of a person who committed suicide will return to exact revenge or achieve redress from those responsible for the suicide (usually abusive in-laws and husbands). The fact that vengeful ghosts and spirits are not mentioned in connection with self-immolations suggests that such acts are not perceived to be ordinary suicides. The spirit of a person who commits suicide out of despair or depression is believed to be intensely dissatisfied and therefore likely to wander as a hungry ghost, whereas self-immolation is believed to be a religious act committed with strong conviction and pure motivation.

Suicide is both a private and social act. Whether it is motivated by despair, religious zeal, or the desire to effect political change, suicide is powerfully symbolic and deeply disturbing. In societies influenced by Chinese culture, individuals are defined within a matrix of family relationships, and because the body is a representation of family continuity, the act of suicide carries a weighty significance. The far-reaching effects of Chinese and Vietnamese self-immolations indicate the power that such actions carry in these family-oriented societies. In a more recent incident in November 1999, Chang Zhichen immolated herself and her infant daughter in Weinan, Shanxi, to protest government persecution of the quasi-Buddhist Falun Gong sect.

Suicide is rare in Tibetan society, so the self-immolation of fifty-year-old Thupten Ngodub, in New Delhi in 1998, had a particularly dramatic impact not just for Tibetans but the international community as well. Despite police and paramilitary troopers who were stationed at the site, Ngodub brought attention to the plight of the Tibetan people by ending a forty-nine-day hunger strike with burning himself to death. His action was motivated by the despair that many Tibetans feel about the fate of their country and their culture under Chinese Communist rule. A statement issued by the Tibetan Youth Congress made clear the intent behind Ngodub's hunger strike and self-immolation: "The Tibetan people have sent a clear message to the world that they can sacrifice themselves for the cause of an independent Tibet. More blood will flow in the coming days. . . . The Tibetan people will fight to the last drop of their blood."[12] This statement supports Sallie B. King's fears that endorsing such acts can precipitate similar acts in the future.[13]

His Holiness the Dalai Lama has consistently eschewed violence in Tibet's struggle for self-determination, but some question the effectiveness of his nonviolent strategy. In an official statement after Ngodub's death, the Dalai Lama expressed his deep sadness at the action. He stated that the protestors acted out of "a sense of frustration and urgency" and were prepared to die "not for their selfish ends but for the rights of six million Tibetans."

King raises important questions about the moral foundation and implications of this antinomian practice among otherwise nonviolent

Buddhists. In a letter to the United States government, Nhat Chi May, a young laywoman and disciple of Thich Nhat Hanh who immolated herself in Saigon in 1967, specifically states that she burned herself for the cause of peace. King believes that May's action was grounded in her spirituality and that she "was acting out of unusually profound faithfulness and obedience to the spiritual principles of her religion."[14] In the Order of Interbeing to which May belonged, however, Thich Nhat Hanh expanded the traditional Vinaya prohibition against taking life to read: "Do not kill. Do not let others kill. Find whatever means possible to protect life and build peace."[15] The traditional precept against taking life or encouraging the taking of life has thus been reinterpreted to include an injunction to prevent others from taking life and to protect life by whatever means possible. This injunction could be taken to mean that suicide is justified to protect the lives of a greater number of beings. King therefore feels that May's self-immolation not only expresses the Buddhist principle of selfless compassion, but also fulfills the mandate of the *Metta Sutta*: "Just as a mother would protect her only child even at the risk of her own life, even so let one cultivate a boundless heart towards all beings."[16]

An act of self-immolation motivated by a desire for nonexistence (*abhaya*) is regarded as a nonvirtuous act of suicide, but an act motivated by the wish to bring peace or save lives may fall in a different category. If the action is taken for the benefit of others and is motivated by the pure thought of compassion, even though negative karma is accrued, the ultimate consequences of the action may be justifiable, even fortunate. The Mahāyāna texts clearly state that an action taken with *bodhicitta*, the altruistic attitude of wishing to achieve enlightenment for the sake of all sentient beings, is infinitely virtuous. In addition, the texts include numerous examples of *bodhisattvas*, including the Buddha in past lives, offering their bodies by fire, by hurling themselves over cliffs, and by feeding their bodies to animals.

The practice of self-immolation raises a number of questions that may have applications for bioethical decision making. First, it raises questions about the motivations that impel human beings to actions of self-sacrifice. The Buddhist emphasis on the role of intention in determining the karmic consequences of an action is well recognized. S. N. Goenka, a well-known Indo-Burmese meditation teacher, illustrates this by juxtaposing the actions of two people who each kill someone with a knife, but for very different reasons. A thief kills a person in the process of a robbery and a doctor kills a patient in the process of an unsuccessful surgery. Both the thief and the doctor kill a human being with a knife, but the motivation behind each of their actions was very different—the thief was motivated by greed, whereas the doctor was motivated by the compassionate wish to save another's life. In the Buddhist interpretation of the law of karma, cause and effect, the results of the two similar actions will be very different. Although the doctor may accumulate a very slight degree of negative karma as a result of killing the patient, it will be insignificant because there was no intention to kill.

It is generally assumed that the motivation for self-immolation in Chinese Buddhist culture is compassion, but other motivations may also be present. There is little reason to doubt that the compassionate acts of *bodhisattvas* recounted in the Buddhist texts are anything but altruistic. For example, there is a Jātaka tale in which Śākyamuni, in a previous life as Mahāsattva, sacrificed his own flesh to prevent a starving tigress from devouring her cubs.[17] However, it is not certain that such passages provided textual justification for the acts of self-sacrifice by Buddhists in China and Vietnam. Buddhists interviewed after self-immolations are of the opinion that, if a person's motivation is not absolutely pure, the pain of autocremation will be unbearable. Not only must one's motivation be pure, but one must also have courage, mental concentration, and strong determination. At least one well-intended self-immolator has been unable to endure the pain.

Second, self-immolation raises the question of quantifying virtue.[18] Can lives be traded on a quid pro quo basis? If sacrificing one life can save five hundred lives, does that numerical ratio change the nature or consequences of a violent act, whether against oneself or another living being? The Mahāyāna *Upāya-kauśalya Sūtra* tells the story of a compassionate ship captain (the Buddha in a past life as a *bodhisattva*) who kills an evil merchant to prevent him from killing 499 other merchants to steal their possessions.[19] This account indicates that a nonvirtuous action may sometimes be justified for the greater good. But calculating the relative merit of actions numerically raises the question of how many lives need to be endangered to justify an act of killing. Further, unless one has supernormal powers, the matter of predicting others' future actions and ascertaining their intentions is highly problematic. In this account, the *bodhisattva*'s action was motivated by pure *bodhicitta* and he presumably possessed the supernormal ability to ascertain the evildoer's intent. Due to his immense compassion, the *bodhisattva*'s action of killing one person to save five hundred is portrayed as justified and the ultimate consequence of his action was a fortunate rebirth. Even then, he was not spared the negative consequences of killing a human being; he had to take birth in a hell realm, though that birth lasted only an instant. This story illustrates that, although the results of negative actions for the benefit of sentient beings may be commuted, a *bodhisattva* must be courageous and compassionate enough to suffer the negative karmic consequences of unwholesome deeds committed for the welfare of sentient beings.

In Buddhist thinking, both actions and motivations are ultimately a matter of personal responsibility, but actions also have social consequences. An act of self-immolation or any other act of self-sacrifice for a good cause may accomplish a constructive aim, but it may also incite others to act similarly, costing numerous lives. King recognizes that, "Each self-immolation moved thousands of people to work to end the war [in Vietnam]," but she also states:

> If the indirect, *but inevitable*, consequence of a self-immolation
> is imitation of the act by others of quite varied motivation,
> then the original self-immolation bears partial karmic respon-
> sibility for those imitations. It must be acknowledged that an
> act that invites other acts of clearly negative karmic and moral
> value cannot itself be cleared of negative moral value.[20]

Buddhists do recognize ethical decisions as matters of both personal and social ethical responsibility, and attempt to resolve problems with compassion and respect for life, but complex ethical dilemmas such as these are rarely discussed. For the most part, Buddhists today are concerned with surviving and with preserving their traditions after suffering tragic losses in the millions as a result of wars and genocide in Cambodia, China, Laos, Mongolia, Tibet, Vietnam, and elsewhere over the last few decades. These tragedies have presented Buddhists with ethical complexities that need to be frankly discussed both within Buddhist institutions, in ecumenical gatherings of Buddhists of different denominations, and in dialogue with other religious traditions. Similar discussions are needed to consider the ethical complexities presented by science and technology.

Pro-life, Pro-choice: Buddhism and Reproductive Ethics

The right to a safe and legal abortion is one of the most volatile and politicized of contemporary ethical issues and the issue is certainly a matter of urgent concern for the world's women. Globally, an estimated 40 percent of two hundred ten million pregnancies each year are unplanned, affecting eighty-four million women and their families. It is estimated that "80,000 women die annually from unsafe abortions" and "15,000 women have abortions each year because they

became pregnant after rape or incest."[21] Feminist theorists suggest that
the criminalization of contraception and abortion is a means of control-
ling women's freedom and power. Although ethical behavior is generally viewed as a means to prevent human suffering, traditional religious
positions about reproductive ethics may also contribute to women's
sufferings by limiting family planning options, as in the example of
preventing artificial birth control. Reproductive ethics involve issues of
sexuality, politics, economics, psychology, gender, and religion, and
evoke a land mine of complex intellectual and emotional responses.

The fact that abortion is mentioned in the earliest strata of Buddhist texts is evidence that abortion has been an issue of human concern for a very long time. In the *Bhikṣuṇī Pratimokṣa Sūtra*, the third
root downfall (*pārājika*) for *bhikṣuṇīs* (fully ordained nuns) specifies
that taking the life of a fetus is taking the life of a human being and
is grounds for expulsion from the order. The precept was created after
it was discovered that a *bhikṣuṇī* had helped a laywoman terminate an
unwanted pregnancy. The commentary on this precept stipulates that
taking the life of a human fetus is taking the life of a human being:
"By the body of a human being is meant that which appears in the
womb of the mother at the time of conception, lasting until the time
of death."[22] Although this precept pertains specifically to *bhikṣuṇīs*, the
prohibition against abortion would similarly apply to a laywoman or
anyone who had taken the precept to refrain from taking life. Even for
those who have not formally taken this precept, to take the life of a
human being is classified as one of the ten nonvirtuous actions
(*daśākuśala*) to be avoided by all decent members of human society.[23]
The texts make no reference to the legal rights of a fetus, but they do
mention that the fetus suffers *in utero*, for example, when the mother
moves suddenly, drinks extremely hot or cold beverages, or engages
in sexual intercourse.

A variety of Buddhist texts and commentaries state that a human
life begins at the moment of conception, which is defined as when the
consciousness of the incipient being enters into the conjoined sperm
and egg of the parents. Because Buddhists regard taking the life of a
fetus or even an embryo as taking the life of a human being, abortion
and other issues of reproductive health raise serious moral, spiritual,
and personal dilemmas. To take the life of a creature belonging to the
animal kingdom is also regarded as unwholesome, but is classified as
a less serious transgression (*pāyantika*).[24] Taking the life of a nonhuman being, such as a demon (*yakṣa*), ghost (*preta*), or animal that has
the power to disguise itself as a human being, is classified as unwholesome, but falls into the less serious category of a fault (*dukkaṭa*).[25]

Because a human lifetime is difficult to obtain, short in duration, and essential for progress on the path to liberation, a human rebirth is regarded as a precious opportunity. On this basis, some Buddhists believe that contraception is ill-advised. For example, there is a Jātaka tale that includes this plea:

> The dew-drop on the blade of grass
> Vanishes when the sun comes up;
> Such is a human span of life;
> So, mother, do not hinder me.[26]

From anecdotal evidence and literary references such as this, it appears that among Buddhists there is a certain bias in favor of conception. Still, there is no textual evidence that preventing conception through such means as artificial contraception is nonvirtuous. In today's world, with tens of millions of women, children, and men suffering from HIV and AIDs, it can be argued that the virtue of compassion makes the use of artificial contraception imperative.

Buddhist texts speak of sentient beings searching for a suitable rebirth, suggesting that the incipient being seeks a couple having sexual relations, which is the door to conception. Family members are thought to have special relationships to each other that are not simply biological, but also the result of karmic affinities, based on close relationships between the mother, father, and child in past lives. In addition to these karmic relationships, parents are thought to have a special responsibility to care for infants, because they are so vulnerable. A mother's relationship to her child is especially valued and is often portrayed as the epitome of human kindness. From evidence in the Vinaya, it is clear that victims of rape are blameless, but many Buddhists would argue in favor of continuing a pregnancy resulting from rape, out of compassion for the incipient child.

The contemporary debate over abortion hinges on determining when life begins. Traditionally, Buddhists assume that the life process of sentient beings born from a womb begins when a being's consciousness "enters" the conjoined egg and sperm of the parents at the moment of conception.[27] Buddhist texts describe conception as occurring at the juncture of three conditions: the unimpaired ovum ("blood") of the mother, the unimpaired sperm of the father, and the "descent" of the incoming being's consciousness into the womb. Although the texts do not specify the precise moment, conception is said to occur when these three conditions converge. This is clear from the rebirth imagery depicted in the Wheel of Life paintings found at the doorway of many (especially Tibetan) Buddhist monasteries. The texts suggest that the consciousness of the incoming being is somehow capable of animating the material elements that constitute a new body, resulting in the generation of a living being. In the twelve links of dependent arising that explain how sentient beings take rebirth, ignorance gives rise to karmic formations, karmic formations give rise to consciousness, consciousness gives rise to name and form, and so on. Consciousness is therefore the activating force that causes sentient beings to come into being. Without consciousness, with merely the genetic components, a living being cannot be said to exist.

Medical science defines conception as fertilization, when the sperm and egg chromosomes fuse together to form the zygote and the new chromosomal arrangement is complete. Medical science also tells us that the process by which the sperm penetrates the outer and inner layers of the ovum can take as long as two to twenty-four hours after intercourse. This information has direct relevance to a discussion of conception and when it occurs. The zygote (the diploid cell resulting from the union of sperm and egg, or fertilized ovum) may then become implanted in the wall of the womb, which occurs up to a week after coitus. The first two weeks after fertilization, sometimes called the pre-embryonic period, characterized by cell division of the zygote. Identical twinning occurs between three and thirteen days after conception; conjoined twinning occurs between thirteen and sixteen days after conception. The moral status of the zygote during the interval between fertilization and implantation (when the fertilized ovum, or blastocyst, attaches to the endometrium of the uterus six or seven days after fertilization) is still a topic of controversy. The precise moment when consciousness enters into this process and the moment when the developing zygote, pre-embryo, embryo, or fetus becomes a person are issues that cannot be addressed by science and require some other rationale.

The world's religious traditions have different theories about when conception occurs and these theories sometimes change over time. The Buddhist texts describe conception as the "descent" of an incipient being who is attracted by desire to the sexual contact of a man and a woman in sexual union. When the consciousness of this being enters into the conjoined sperm of the father and egg of the mother, conception occurs. The moment of conception is also sometimes called "re-becoming" or "re-linking"; some Tibetan texts refer to it as the *bardo* of becoming. The traditional Buddhist explanation of conception resembles fertilization, but does not take into account the time that elapses between the penetration of the ovum by the sperm and the final fusing of the male and female chromosomes during the process of fertilization. It also does not take into account the possibility of identical or conjoined twins forming during the "preembryonic" period when the cells of the zygote divide, or the time lapse before implantation. In any case, traditionally Buddhists believe that a sentient being exists from the moment the consciousness enters into the conjoined sperm and egg.

The Vinaya texts provide the theoretical framework for Buddhist ethics and serve as a reference point for examining questions of bioethics. Damien Keown comments that the early Buddhists, particularly monks, tended to dissociate themselves from questions of sexuality and reproduction,[28] but the discussions of sexual matters in the Vinaya are remarkably frank. The precepts or regulations found in the Vinaya evolved gradually, on a case by case basis as problematic situations arose. Some of the cases that served as precedents for the creation of particular precepts included some very bawdy behavior. Complaints were brought to the attention of the Buddha, who called the accused to explain the situation and then made a ruling that applied henceforth to all monks and, subsequently, nuns. After a ruling was made, modifications were often created for exceptional circumstances. The Vinaya regulations serve as a basis of interpretation in assessing cases for which there is no textual precedent. This process of interpolating from the existing precepts to evaluate new situations is sanctioned in the final instructions that the Buddha gave just before he passed away:

> Practice whatever is in accordance
> with what I have allowed;
> Abandon whatever is in accordance
> with what I have prohibited.[29]

For example, the texts do not mention contemporary family planning methods that prevent conception. Based on similar dilemmas and decisions described in the texts, one can surmise that contraceptives that prevent conception are allowable, since they do not destroy life that has already begun. One can similarly surmise that contraceptives that terminate a pregnancy are not allowable, since they are thought to destroy life that has already begun. When asked about contraception, Dr. Yeshi Donden, a traditionally trained Tibetan doctor practicing in Dharamsala, explains a commonly accepted view:

> Contraception is not so bad from the point of view of religion [Dharma], because you are not killing anyone. Even though contraception stops someone from coming into the

> womb, you would not be throwing anyone out who had
> already gotten into the womb and so you do not have the
> fault of murder. Still, you would have the lesser fault of not
> allowing the consciousness to enter the womb. If you take
> medicine in order to expel a child that has formed in the
> womb, that has the greater fault of committing murder.[30]

Expelling a fetus from the womb is clearly considered nonvirtuous,
but the point at which an embryo becomes a viable fetus is unclear.

For Buddhists, life is presumed to begin at the moment of conception, when the consciousness enters the meeting of the egg of the
mother and the sperm of the father. The passages in the Vinaya that
proscribe abortion specifically refer to a fetus, which is thought to
have consciousness and therefore to be a sentient being. The claim
that a human fetus is a sentient being is based on the supposition that
it possesses the five aggregates that are the basis for imputing the
existence of a person. This would indicate sometime between the third
and the eighth week of embryonic development, when the cardiovas-
cular and neurological systems begin to form. Even though the faculties of an embryo or a fetus are not fully developed, beings at this state
of development have traditionally been regarded as sentient life and
capable of feeling. A question remains, however, about whether there
is a difference between an abortion performed in the first trimester
and one performed in the second or third trimester. It is not easy to
ascertain whether or when an embryo or a fetus possesses all the five
aggregates, but traditionally the presence of consciousness has been
the minimal criterion for determining the presence of a sentient being.
If it can be demonstrated that fertilization can occur without the ingress of a consciousness, it may be possible for the biological conditions for life to be present (a fertilized embryo) without the life of a
sentient being commencing. This question becomes important when
examining issues of *in vitro* fertilization and stem cell research.

From a Buddhist point of view, the genetic components of a
human being alone, absent consciousness, are an insufficient basis for
the existence of a sentient being. Damien Keown assumes that during
in vitro fertilization, consciousness joins the genetic components, but
his conclusion ignores the emotional component of conception. In explaining the process of conception, certain Buddhist texts state that the
bardo being is attracted by sexual desire to the parents in coitus, specifically to the parent of the opposite gender. Thus, the element of
sexual desire is a necessary impetus for fertilization to occur. Contrar-
ily, if a being has eliminated desire, it is possible to avoid taking

rebirth. The *Sūtra of Teaching to Nanda on Entry to the Womb* describes the process by which the *bardo* being (also referred to as a *gandharva*, or smell eater) enters the mother's womb:

> A smell-eater who has these six conditions[31] sees in an illusory manner the father and mother lying together. Due to wanting to copulate, if it is to be reborn as a male, it desires the mother and wishes to separate from the father; whereas, if it is to be reborn as a female, it desires the father and wishes to separate from the mother. Then, when it begins to embrace the one that is desired, through the force of previous actions it does not perceive any part of the body except the person's sexual organ, whereby anger is generated. This desire and hatred act as the cause of death, and the intermediate being enters the womb.[32]

Some Buddhist philosophical and medical literature describe, in remarkable if technically inaccurate detail, the stages of development of the embryo and fetus month by month, sometimes accompanied by illustrations.[33] In addition to the developing aggregate of form, a fetus is said to have the aggregates of feeling (heat, cold, pain, discomfort), perception (of being cramped, bounced, and restricted), karmic formations (for example, the *vāsanā*, imprints of actions or "seeds"), and consciousness (the momentary mental continuum that is imbued with the imprints of actions). As a result of previous skillful or unskillful actions, the being possesses certain predispositions. For example, the being may be predisposed to a longer or shorter life span, to be studious or frivolous, shy or outgoing, loving or aggressive, and so forth. Presently Dr. Ming T. Tsuang, a genetic psychiatrist at Harvard and UCSD, is conducting research to determine whether human qualities such as kindness and compassion may have a genetic component. From a Buddhist standpoint, it is natural that people have specific predispositions as a result of their actions in past lives, though these tendencies are also modified by education and other life experiences.

Buddhist texts treat a fetus as a human being and regard taking the life of a fetus as equivalent to taking the life of a human being, but do not answer the question of whether the action becomes more unwholesome as the fetus grows. The texts also do not discuss abortion in extenuating circumstances such as rape, incest, severe congenital deformity, or cases of mental, physical, or emotional abuse. His Holiness the fourteenth Dalai Lama has taken an active interest in medical research that might bear on the question of precisely when consciousness enters a fertilized ovum. As discussed earlier, if consciousness enters at the moment of conception, then methods of terminating pregnancy after the moment of conception would constitute taking life. If consciousness enters the embryo at some later time, it would not. This determination has been hindered by the difficulty of scientifically defining and measuring consciousness. If science could verify that the consciousness does not enter the developing embryo until the heartbeat and brain waves are detectable during the fourth week, then Buddhists would have cause to review and perhaps revise their stance on abortion.

In 1992, the Dalai Lama voiced the unorthodox and controversial view that there may be situations in which abortion may be warranted, such as when a fetus is so severely damaged that it would endure great suffering throughout its life. However, the decision to abort a severely disabled fetus may be motivated by factors other than compassion; social, psychological, and economic factors may also be involved. The Dalai Lama has continued to gather information from the medical and scientific communities to broaden his understanding of the complex issues involved, but thus far he has upheld the traditional view—that abortion involves taking the life of a sentient being and is a seriously unwholesome action.

From a Buddhist point of view, the decision to terminate a pregnancy is an enormous ethical responsibility that involves not only the immediate welfare of both fetus and family members in this life, but in future lives as well. Although the process of rebirth is beyond ordinary beings' capacity to perceive, every action is said to set in motion a string of consequences that then serve as the conditions for future actions. The quality of each action and the intention behind it not only shape one's present identity, but also affect one's innumerable future identities and circumstances. Each action creates its own momentum either toward liberation or toward the continual sufferings of circling within *saṃsāra*. Every action is therefore pivotal in one's future evolution and deserves careful reflection.

To date, many of the studies on Buddhism and abortion have focused on Japan, especially the ritual known as *mizuko kuyō* and its American adaptations.[34] Because reliable methods of contraception were not readily available in Japan until recently, abortion became the principal means of birth control for Japanese women, many of whom have undergone as many as six or more abortions. The *mizuko* ritual is widely performed for commercial gain and has been criticized as exploitative to women, but it is also a way for women to cope with the grief, loss, and shame they feel as a consequence of having an abortion.[35] In this ritual, one who has experienced abortion or the loss of a child may pray to Jizō Bodhisattva, who is regarded as a protector of women and children, and transfer the merit accumulated through prayer to comfort the spirit of the departed. In recent years in Japan, a schedule of fees for this ritual service has replaced the donation system and dealing with the regrets that often attend abortion has become big business. Unscrupulous entrepreneurs have taken advantage of women by raising the specter of harmful influences from the vengeful spirits of *mizuko*, then charging dearly for rites to propitiate and exorcize these spirits. There is little doubt that commercialization of the *mizuko kuyō* by certain opportunistic temples and entrepreneurs has undermined Buddhism's moral authority in Japan, at least to some extent, regardless of wide social acceptance of abortion as a "necessary sorrow."

Japanese *mizuko kuyō* beliefs and practices have no textual source in the Buddhist canon and are in no way typical of practices in other Buddhist countries and cultures. Nevertheless, as William R. LaFleur notes, in Japan these rituals have become an important means for women to come to terms with their decision to terminate a pregnancy:

> Thus, parental prayers and ritual memorializations were expected to palliate guilt, create what is taken to be a continuing relationship between parents in this world and a fetus in a Buddhist "limbo," and render close to moot many of the West's protracted debates about life's inception, fetal rights, and ownership of the bodies of women.[36]

There is a widespread belief in many modern cultures that abortion is necessary for the health of society, for reasons that go beyond the scope of this study. In Japan, the practice of abortion is justified by an unusual, somewhat naïve interpretation of Buddhist doctrine:

> ... [H]istorically the belief in transmigration and rebirth effectively attenuated any sense of "finality" in abortion— thus giving the "parents" of an aborted fetus the expectation that the fetus' entry into the world had been merely postponed.[37]

This interpretation avoids some important questions about karmic retribution. There is also a danger that this logic could be used to rid society of the old, sick, dying, criminal, or socially disruptive.

Robert Aitken, a well-known American Zen master, created a Buddhist ritual both to mourn the loss of an aborted fetus and to comfort parents who had made such a tragic decision.[38] Yvonne Rand, a Sōtō Zen priest trained at the San Francisco Zen Center, has adapted the *mizuko* ritual to help American women come to terms with the grief and trauma they often experience from the loss of a child in an accident or an abortion, whether spontaneous or induced. Each woman sews a bib and offers it to an image of Jizō Bodhisattva with prayers for the well-being of the child. Although there is concern, both in Japan and the United States, that the ritual may be interpreted as condoning abortion or providing a kind of penance, it has proved to be an effective way for women to deal with the psychological effects of abortion.[39] Meditations on loving kindness and compassion for oneself, the aborted fetus or child, and all sentient beings help to replace feelings of sadness and depression.

The debate over abortion raises questions about conflicting rights as well as conflicting values. The argument that a woman has a right to abortion by virtue of owning her body is difficult to reconcile with Buddhist ways of thinking.[40] Buddhist texts and teachers speak of the mother's kindness in bringing a child to term, enduring the pain of giving birth to a child, and coping with the hardships involved in raising a child, but they do not speak in terms of ownership. The mother's personhood is adduced on the basis of her physicality and mentality, and the personhood of the fetus is adduced in a similar manner, so there are no grounds to assume that the mother's claim to life is greater than the child's. Each human life is regarded as the fortunate result of an enormous accumulation of merit over many lifetimes and there is no assurance that another human opportunity will come again any time soon. Therefore the fetus has an equal claim to life and to arbitrate between competing claims to life is an enormous responsibility. Life is a value rather than a right, and to protect life is a primary virtue.

One problem with the rights argument is that it assumes that there is a solid person to whom rights attach. Because there is no truly existent person, the notion of "owning" one's body does not arise. Buddhists may accept the view that one has the right to do with the body as one pleases, but with the understanding that certain consequences are entailed. Another problem with the rights argument is the extent of personal rights. In current discussions of human rights, a discourse strongly influenced by Western thought, the referent is assumed to be solid and inviolable but this assumption does not hold in Buddhist ethics. For example, in a case where the mother's life will be endangered by the birth of a child, a traditional Buddhist perspective would value the two lives equally, rather than assuming that the mother owns her body and that her claim is greater than the child's. Even if the decision is made to save the mother's life at the expense of the child's, it will not be because the child is less equally human. When the reason for seeking abortion is anything less than the life of the mother, then the equation shifts, since it means weighing a human life against something of lesser value. Buddhist texts do not calculate human life in this way. Although human life may be valued more highly than animal life, the first precept clearly treats taking the life of a fetus and an adult as equally censurable.

In sum, the principle values in Buddhist ethics are harmlessness (*ahiṃsā*), wishing to alleviate the sufferings of living beings (*karuṇā*), and wishing to bring happiness to living beings (*maitrī*). But Buddhists acknowledge the impossibility of avoiding the taking of life altogether. They recognize that even the plowing and sowing necessary to maintain a vegetarian diet unavoidably take the lives of many insects. Again, intention is seen as the crucial factor. Actions motivated by compassion will yield different results than those motivated by greed, hatred, and ignorance. But these general principles are inadequate to resolve a moral dilemma like abortion, for both the act of abortion and the act of preventing abortion can result in great suffering for both parents and fetus. Traditionally, reproductive health education has not been the responsibility of Buddhist educators, but Buddhist ethics can be utilized to address these quandaries in society today. Since contraception is allowable, then mindfulness practice can help prevent unwanted pregnancies, and when unwanted pregnancies do occur, Buddhist meditations on compassion can be useful for all concerned. Advocating respect both for life and for the rights of human beings to make their own ethical choices is consistent with Buddhist principles.

Buddhism and Organ Transplantation

The practice of donating one's vital organs for medical research or for transplantation by surgical means has become increasingly common in recent decades, but the ethical issues raised by the practice have yet to be thoroughly discussed in Buddhist circles. In conversations with Buddhists of various backgrounds, most respondents spontaneously supported the idea of donating one's vital organs to save someone's life as consistent with Buddhist values of generosity and loving kindness. Followers of the Theravāda and the Japanese Zen tradition emphasized that, from a Buddhist point of view, the body is merely a collection of disposable parts that has no usefulness after death. The body will be burned or will decompose after we die anyway, so why not use it to benefit others? They believed that a person's consciousness leaves the body at the time of death, so there is no harm in touching, washing, or cutting the body. A person after death is just a corpse—a heap of dead skin, bones, flesh, and other components destined to disintegrate. In Theravāda Buddhist cultures, it is nevertheless customary to wash the body, dress it in fresh clothes, and leave it lying in state for some time (usually one to three days) until the time of cremation. These customs vary depending on the locality, the status of the deceased, the climate, and the wishes of survivors.

Mahāyāna informants have tended to emphasize the value of human life for spiritual practice. Because a human rebirth is difficult to attain, highly perishable, and essential for progressing on the path to enlightenment, practitioners regarded organ donation as an excellent way to create merit through the practice of compassion. To donate a vital organ gives another person the chance to have a longer life and to use it meaningfully for Dharma practice. After death, one's vital organs are no longer useful, so they may as well be used to benefit others. As one bumper sticker reads: "Recycle yourself. Be an organ donor." Organ donation is considered a valuable opportunity on several levels. First, to donate one's body for research or organ transplantation is a way to sever attachment to one's own body. Second, to place another person's welfare above one's own is a perfect expression of the *bodhisattva* ethic of compassion. Third, to donate one's organs with the pure motivation to benefit others will bring great fruits of merit in future lives, enabling one to gain a fortunate rebirth and further opportunities for Dharma practice; if the gift is dedicated to the enlightenment of all beings, the fruits are immeasurable. Buddhist informants from a wide variety of ethnicities and traditions stressed the power of an organ donor's motivation. To donate them for the sake of money or reputation is a defiled motivation.

The selfless *bodhisattva* is esteemed in all Buddhist traditions and taken as a model of compassionate self-sacrifice by Mahāyāna practitioners in particular. Out of great compassion, the *bodhisattva* renounces self-concern and pledges to become a perfectly awakened Buddha in order to liberate all beings from suffering. With that noble aim, the *bodhisattva* postpones final awakening and deliberately takes rebirth for three countless aeons in order to accumulate the wisdom and merit needed to become a Buddha. Working through ten stages (*bhūmis*) of practicing the ten perfections, the *bodhisattva* willingly endures unimaginable hardships in the service of sentient beings, even making sacrifices of the flesh to relieve these beings' hunger.[41] The *bodhisattva's* courage is a model of the selfless resolve and unwavering concentration that a dying individual needs to obtain an excellent rebirth and for an organ donor to accomplish a flawless act of generosity.

Although taking the life of a sentient being, especially a human being, violates a cardinal principle of Buddhist ethics, to sacrifice oneself with the *bodhicitta* motivation of wishing to establish all beings in a state of perfect enlightenment is considered praiseworthy. Narratives of the Buddha's exemplary sacrifices and heroism in his past lives as a *bodhisattva* are preserved in the popular Jātaka tales. The story mentioned earlier of the *bodhisattva* offering flesh from his thigh to save a hungry tigress and her cubs from starvation is widely known in Buddhist cultures and is commemorated at a spot called Namo Buddha in Nepal. The Buddha's sacrifice is mentioned in the liturgy of the *chö* ritual, in which Tibetan practitioners symbolically sacrifice their body parts as a way to cut through attachment and cultivate the perfection of generosity:

> When he was born as King Great and Powerful Compassion
> He fed the tigress with his own flesh.
> In the same way, may I be able to give with joy
> This cherished illusory body to the host of flesh-eaters.[42]

Another example of self-sacrifice is the story of the famed Buddhist saint Asaṅga who cut flesh from his own body to entice maggots away from the vermin-infested body of a dying dog. As a result of this act of compassion, Asaṅga was rewarded by a direct vision of Mañjuśrī.

Whether actual or symbolic, such acts of sacrifice are not to be taken lightly. Without strong and unwavering resolve, one might fall prey to fear and regret. This is illustrated by the story of a demon (*rakṣa*) who cunningly tested a practitioner's resolve. When asked for his eyes, the practitioner plucked them out without hesitation. When asked for his right arm, he sawed it off and offered that, too. When he offered his right arm with his left (unclean) hand, the only one he had left, though, the demon got angry. At this, the practitioner lost his temper and thereby destroyed all the roots of merit he had accumulated through his generosity. This story demonstrates that sacrificing one's life is virtuous when performed with pure motivation, but it requires tremendous determination, discipline, and courage.

In cultures influenced by Confucian thought, there is a traditional aversion to cutting, burning, or violating a corpse in any way. Burial is generally preferred over cremation, since to intentionally damage the integrity of the body bequeathed by the ancestors is regarded as unfilial. For this reason, instances of sacrificing the body, such as by self-immolation, have an especially powerful impact. Occasionally young monks or nuns burn off one or more fingers as an offering to the Buddha and a symbol of their dedication to the welfare of sentient beings. Even today, candidates at Chinese and Korean Buddhist *bodhisattva* ordination ceremonies burn small cones of incense on their scalp or arm to symbolize their willingness to work for the welfare of sentient beings. This custom has no Buddhist antecedent and may simply have been a device to distinguish genuine monks from criminals hiding out in the monasteries, but it has become a way to demonstrate one's commitment to liberating sentient beings. The discomfort pales compared to the *bodhisattva*'s resolve to enter the lowest hells to rescue even one sentient being from suffering. The ritual signifies that the *bodhisattva*'s compassion extends beyond his or her own family to the entire human family and all living beings.

Overall, the intent to donate one's body parts to charity is congruent with the Buddhists' compassionate ideal. It meets with resistance only in those cultures influenced by the Confucian reluctance to disfigure the body. This reluctance accounts for the relatively low rate of organ donors in East Asian societies. Attitudes are changing, but the State of Hawai'i, with its large Asian population, still has the lowest rate of organ donations in the United States. Recent efforts by Buddhists to encourage organ donation in Korea and Taiwan have been remarkably successful, however. In all these cases, it is assumed that an organ donor is motivated purely by the thought to benefit, not money or reputation.

Two questions remain that may cause Buddhists to hesitate in agreeing to organ donation. First, if the organs must be harvested before the vital signs cease, this will cause the death of the patient, which is unfortunate for both the medical technician and the patient. Second, even if the organs are harvested after the vital signs cease, the procedure may disturb the dying person's consciousness and lead to an unfortunate rebirth. One's state of mind during the process of dying is of crucial importance for determining one's future rebirth. Ridding oneself of personal attachments and antipathies before the time of death helps make the transition to the next life easier. Prayers may be offered to benefit the deceased in the next life. To die in an angry state of mind, on the other hand, can lead to a hellish rebirth. Manuals such as *Liberation by Hearing in the Intermediate State* (*Bar do tho drol*) describe the terrifying visions and sensations a person may experience during the dying process and provide instructions about how to traverse the intermediate state without fear, anger, or trepidation. With such manuals as a guide, practitioners can train their minds beforehand and prepare themselves to die intelligently and consciously.

Both Theravāda and Mahāyāna Buddhists generally believe that it is best to avoid disturbing a person during the dying process. The idea is to create a calm atmosphere so that the dying person can single-pointedly concentrate on the stages of the dying process. In Buddhist societies, a terminally ill patient may be advised to give away all possessions before the time of death, both to circumvent attachment to the objects and to create merit for a better rebirth. It is especially important that loved ones refrain from crying, arguing, or otherwise troubling the dying person's mind. If loved ones are calm, authentic, and loving, they can be a comforting presence at the bedside. Other-wise, if they may cause attachment or unease to arise in the mind of the dying person, it is better for loved ones to chant, pray, or simply generate loving thoughts from another room.[43] Unless the dying person has been a serious practitioner and liberation is at hand, the time has come for one existence to end and another one to begin, so it is essential that the person avoid clinging to the things of this life.

As death nears, Tibetans avoid unnecessarily touching or disturbing the body in any way. It is especially important to avoid touching the lower extremities, because this may cause the consciousness to exit from the lower part of the body and therefore be drawn to rebirth in a lower realm. It is also vital to avoid inciting emotions such as greed, attachment, and especially anger in the dying person at all costs. As far as possible, it is best to leave the body alone and in quietude for two or three days after the pulse and breathing have stopped, or until the corpse begins to decompose. When the body begins to emit a foul odor, it is a sure sign that the consciousness is no longer present. In some cases, a white drop will appear at the area of the nostrils. To interrupt the dying process before this time is po-tentially disruptive to the dying person's subtle consciousness and may be detrimental to the person's future state of rebirth.

If we accept the possibility that an individual's mental con-tinuum does not cease when the respiration and pulse stop but continues on through the *bardo* and another rebirth, then Buddhists are faced with a dilemma. On the one hand, the physical aggregates are useless after death and to donate one's eyes, liver, kidneys, or other organs is a greatly compassionate act. On the other hand, to ensure a positive rebirth for the benefit of oneself and others, the dying person must not be disturbed. For organ donation to be suc-cessful, however, the process of harvesting the organs must begin immediately after clinical death. A heart that has ceased functioning may be useless, so the surgical removal must take place immediately upon death or even before. Unless a person is extremely well-trained, the consciousness is likely to be disturbed by the surgery and it may be best to avoid organ transplantation. A *bodhisattva* may have the steadiness of concentration and depth of compassion to remain unperturbed during the extraction of the vital organs, but an ordinary person without steady concentration and unwavering compassion may be vulnerable to anger at that moment and thereby risk a disastrous rebirth.

When I asked Lama Karma Rinchen, spiritual director of Kagyu Thekchen Ling, a Tibetan Buddhist center in Honolulu, whether he thought it was a good idea to donate one's organs at the time of death, he immediately answered in the affirmative. "Definitely," he said, "That is an excellent compassionate *bodhisattva* action." When I asked him whether the dying person's consciousness would be disturbed by getting an organ cut out, he said, "That's okay. The doctors can wait for a few days." When I explained that the doctors have to remove the organ immediately in order to save the life of the recipient, he expressed alarm. After some reflection, he concluded that for an ordinary person who believes that the mind dies with the body, it is fine to donate one's organs, but for a Buddhist practitioner, it might be better to wait until the *bodhisattva* resolve is unshakeable. Despite the risk, out of compassion, he personally plans to donate his organs anyway.

The issue of organ donation raises many psychological, philosophical, and economic issues, too numerous to review here. Buddhist responses to these issues also vary widely, according to the teacher and the tradition. A primary consideration is whether or not an organ donor's life is terminated prematurely in order to ensure a successful transplant. If so, the issue is clearly more complex than a simple trade of one life for another, even if the donor is the victim of a serious accident with no chance for survival. To ensure a successful transplant, a donated heart must be surgically removed while it is still beating, yet this removal also results in the death of the donor. The ramifications of prematurely removing organs are not far to see. Hence, there has been considerable debate about the ethics of extracting the organs of anencephalic infants for immediate use, rather than waiting for death to occur, based on the view that these infants lack substantial higher cognitive functions. The ethics of organ transplantation therefore requires careful consideration of many issues, including the criteria for determining the death of the human organism, the ethics of prolonging life artificially, the ethics of withdrawing extraordinary life-support measures, psychological concerns, economic concerns such as allocation of resources, and culturally diverse definitions of death with dignity.

In making decisions about organ transplantation, determining the moment of death is medically, morally, and legally significant.

Criteria such as the cessation of the vital signs and brain death may be inadequate for determining the moment of death. Because all organ systems fail when brain function stops, and the individual stands no chance of recovery or of leading a "meaningful" life, a diagnosis of brain death is regarded as sufficient justification for withdrawing extraordinary life-support measures and for permitting the surgical removal of organs for transplantation. From a Tibetan Buddhist perspective, however, it is the experience of the clear light that is the factor that determines the death of an individual and any intervention before that time, especially in the case of a skilled meditation practitioner, is inadvisable. Furthermore, debates about the ethics of organ transplantation have revealed that modern medical methods of prolonging life are also becoming methods of prolonging death. For Buddhists, the ethics of organ transplantation raises questions that go beyond the scope of traditional injunctions and meditations for mindful dying. In order to make well-informed decisions about such issues as organ donation, Buddhists need to gain greater familiarity with medical procedures and practices, and engage in thorough reflection and dialogue on Buddhist determinations of the moment of death.

Chapter 9

Extending Life
and Hastening Death

In recent years, the topics of euthanasia and assisted suicide have become the focus of much heated debate. Now that medically extending life and deciding on a time to die have become options, the questions of whether and how long to live have become highly charged ethical and social concerns. Although the option of extending life technologically is still not open for terminally ill patients in most parts of the world, it has become the prerogative of a privileged segment of the world's population—those who live in developed countries and have means and access to advanced medical technologies. Societies with the most advanced medical technologies also happen to have the most rapidly aging populations. It is probably not surprising that several end-of-life cases, particularly in the United States, have become the focus of public debate.

To better understand this emotionally charged debate, it is necessary to distinguish between the terms euthanasia and assisted suicide, both active and passive, voluntary and involuntary. The word *euthanasia* derives from two Greek roots and can be translated as "good death."[1] Originally associated with the voluntary drinking of hemlock to painlessly escape the suffering of sickness and aging, the term gradually came to be applied to a physician's means of hastening death.[2] The term is often glossed as mercy killing or compassionate murder, though these interpretations are not universally accepted, as we shall see.

According to Tom L. Beauchamp's evaluation, active euthanasia involves "the act or practice of intentionally, mercifully, and painlessly causing the death of persons suffering from serious injuries, system failures, or fatal diseases. Here the emphasis is on acting rather than omitting to act, suggesting killing rather than allowing a death to occur."[3] Passive euthanasia involves "failing to prevent death from natural causes in cases of terminal illness."[4] With advances in medical technology since the 1970s, passive euthanasia has increasingly come to mean withdrawing extraordinary means of preserving life but, by this definition, it could also include not seeking medical means of extending life. When euthanasia is requested by the patient, it is termed "voluntary." An example of voluntary euthanasia is when a patient suffering severely from a terminal illness gradually stops eating or takes an overdose of barbituates and dies. When euthanasia is not requested by the patient, due to mental incompetence or some other debility, it is termed "involuntary."[5] An example of involuntary euthanasia is when a physician or caregiver, out of compassion, withholds nutrition or administers an overdose of barbituates to a mentally incapacitated patient suffering severely from a terminal illness, and the patient dies. In assisted suicide the death is caused by the patient's action, whereas in voluntary active euthanasia the death is caused by another person's action. Despite the usefulness of distinguishing these categories, however, it must be recognized that the lines between euthanasia, suicide, and assisted suicide, whether active or passive, voluntary or involuntary, cannot always be sharply drawn.

Beauchamp specifies three necessary characteristics of euthanasia: (1) at least one other person is involved in intending and causing the patient's death; (2) the primary consideration for intending the patient's death is to end acute suffering or an irreversible comatose condition; and (3) the means of death is as painless as possible (unless moral justification exists for another method).[6] Physician-assisted suicide is often regarded as a form of voluntary active euthanasia, but there is a distinction. In the case of euthanasia, the patient is often in great pain and the method chosen to terminate life is to relieve the patient's suffering as painlessly as possible. In the case of assisted suicide, the patient is not necessarily suffering acutely and the means of death is not necessarily the most painless. Some believe that euthanasia is warranted only in the case of a diagnosed incurable terminal illness; others believe that euthanasia is justified for other mentally or physically debilitating conditions as well.

In recent years, in relation to new medical technologies, there has been a shift toward greater precision in defining the boundaries between euthanasia, suicide, assisted suicide, and withdrawal of treatment. A careful delineation of these terms presupposes a system of medical technology capable of diagnosing terminal illness and a society where medical professionals are entrusted with life and death decisions. At the same time, there is a growing recognition that caregivers other than medical professionals may also be involved. Important questions remain about what constitutes due process in making decisions about the termination of life, the effectiveness of pain management, and issues about dosages of pain medication.

In an analysis of Hindu attitudes toward euthanasia, Katherine K. Young uses the ancient Greek definition, "freedom to leave," and applies it to an analysis of euthanasia in classical India. Since Vedic times, Indian society has been decidedly life affirming, with an ideal life span of "one hundred autumns." Despite Indian society's strong valuation of long life, however, Young identifies three categories of culturally accepted self-willed death in the Brahmanical context: suicide resulting from depression and melancholy; heroic voluntary death to avoid capture, rape, or slavery; and religious self-willed death by fasting (*prāyopaveśana*). The latter practice is similar to *sallekhanā*, the religious practice of abstaining from nutrition and hydration, that is esteemed among the Jains.[7]

The practice of fasting at the end of life is not limited to India, of course. Like other animals, people often stop taking food and water toward the end of their lives. To stop eating is a natural reaction for many human beings when their energy is declining and their digestion failing. In the Tibetan texts that describe the signs of the dissolution of the elements of the body during the process of dying, the gradual failure of the digestive processes signals the dissolution of the fire element. Questions about whether a death resulting from a voluntary failure to take food or water is morally significant or whether such a death is a type of suicide are among the many ethical ambiguities that are still open for consideration.

The Ethics of Extending Life

The human desire for longevity is universal and easily understandable. From a Buddhist perspective, however, longevity is not universally beneficial. Buddhists contend that long life is desirable for the virtuous, but undesirable for the nonvirtuous. A murderer who is unrepentant and continually kills, for example, is constantly accumulating nonvirtuous karma, which is harmful to both the murderer and others. Unless the person is contrite and renounces such serious wrongdoing, it would be better to have a short life span. Buddhists apply this reasoning only to a natural death, of course, and do not use it to justify the premature termination of the murderer's life span. The statement that a short lifetime is better for the nonvirtuous may be didactic, calculated to deter wrongdoing and reduce suffering all the way around. By the same token, it is said that a virtuous person profits from a long life span, by having more time to accumulate good deeds. This naturally appeals to human beings' desire for life and inspires them to mental cultivation and accumulation of merit. For Buddhists, these pursuits—mental cultivation and the accumulation of merit—are the gauge for assessing the quality of a life. Buddhists commonly exhort one another to make life meaningful with adages such as, "Human life is precious, not to be squandered."

For Buddhists, a meaningful life is one that is rich in virtue or merit. The quality of a person's life has little to do with such indicators as health, beauty, productivity, or freedom from pain, except insofar as they inhibit one's ability to create virtue. The frail, elderly, and terminally ill may not be productive in terms of worldly accomplishments and the market economy, but they can still practice virtue, which in any case is regarded as the best use of a person's time and the best way to achieve both immediate happiness and a fortunate rebirth. Merit does not necessarily require physical agility or strength, but can also be accumulated through generating virtuous thoughts. There is a story about a wealthy benefactor who offered a sumptuous feast to the Buddha and his entourage. As the Buddha and his disciples arrived, they noticed a poor man sitting outside the gate. After the sumptuous meal, the benefactor asked who accumulated the most merit that day, expecting praise for his generosity. The Buddha replied that the poor man sitting outside the gate had accumulated the most merit that day. The benefactor was furious, because he had gone to considerable expense and effort, and demanded an explanation. The Buddha replied that, although the poor man had nothing material to offer, he had accumulated an immense store of merit simply by rejoicing in the benefactor's merit, without any expectation of praise or reward. Generating thoughts of generosity is an exceptional way to create merit.

Old age can be an excellent time for spiritual practice, because there are fewer distractions and demands on one's time. Physical disabilities or weakness need not diminish a person's sense of worth or capacity to be spiritually productive. On the contrary, reflections on the frailty of the human body and the sufferings of living beings are time-honored Buddhist methods of contemplation. The end of life can be viewed as a special opportunity to generate thoughts of loving kindness and compassion for all those beings who are beset by the sufferings that attend old age and death. Buddhist meditation methods not only provide myriad ways of cultivating the mind, but are also ideal means of achieving tranquility, contentment, and mental alertness at a most opportune juncture. Being old and fragile can engender a deep empathy for the anxieties and sufferings of others. Instead of growing resentful of the limitations aging brings or wasting time in senseless activities, the frail and elderly can transform the experience of aging and the immanence of dying into a vital spiritual practice.

Buddhist cultures offer a wealth of practical methods for coping with death. Reflection on suffering and impermanence helps one develop insight into the universality of these experiences. Reflecting on the law of cause and effect, regretting all misdeeds, and rejoicing in the virtuous actions of oneself and others engenders equanimity and inner peace. Understanding the workings of cause and effect helps one accept sickness, suffering, and death, not as a punishment, but as the natural course of events in *saṃsāra*. This naturally leads to a sense of acceptance of one's own death. Reflecting on the virtue of generosity inspires one to distribute one's wealth before the moment of death. The practice of generosity not only generates merit, but it also engenders detachment, and this practice of letting go makes dying easier. The practice of generosity accumulates merit, brings happiness to both the giver and receiver, and benefits society by reapportioning wealth and alleviating poverty. Instead of feeling alienated, lonely, and helpless, these simple practices help even the most debilitated person to live meaningfully up until the very moment of death. The belief that the virtue accrued in this lifetime brings happiness in the future helps overcome the fear of death.

Nurses who work in hospices and emergency rooms often hear patients regret the way they have lived. Buddhist repentance practices are a way to deal with regret and to use one's time wisely to create merit. From a Buddhist perspective, caregivers and medical personnel also create great merit by being loving, kind, and attentive to patients' needs. Compassionate healthcare and spiritual care, along with adequate pain medication, help diminish people's feelings of despair and the desire to end life.

Arguing For and Against Euthanasia

End-of-life decision making may have been easier in earlier times when the majority of people relied on the authority of religious beliefs passed down through generations and had fewer options regarding when and how to die. The received wisdom of tradition was more universally accepted and was a nonnegotiable set of cultural values that guided ethical decision making, interpersonal relations, and even the way a person would psychologically approach problem solving. In recent years, a variety of factors has made life more complex: the influence of secularization, changing lifestyles, longer life spans, enhanced medical technologies, the high cost of medical care, and the vast array of available lifestyle choices. In view of all these complex factors, a groundswell in favor of decriminalizing euthanasia has gained momentum, inciting an equally strong force to oppose it.

Advocates on both sides advance their arguments for and against euthanasia and assisted suicide. Proponents invoke the rights of human beings to decide for themselves when and how to end their days on Earth. Many appeal for compassion in supporting the rights of severely disabled patients to die on their own terms. Opponents invoke the sanctity of life and divine authority in matters of life and death. There are legitimate fears that the right to terminate one's own life may lead to abuses to the detriment of the aging, disabled, and dying. Many argue that better patient care would alleviate the feelings of hopelessness, burdensomeness, and despair that often arise among the disabled and terminally ill. At the same time, better patient care has resulted in more complicated care problems, including multiple conditions (diabetes, stroke side effects, incontinence, adverse drug interactions, and so on) affecting a single patient. There are also many people who feel ambivalent, conflicted, or uncomfortable about weighing in on the potential abuses or benefits of the right to decide one's own time of death.

Generally speaking, most societies regard the taking of human life as morally repugnant. This stance is strongly reinforced by religious tenets, legal codes, and social taboos in almost all cultures. Despite the fact that human blood is shed in enormous quantities in senseless wars, criminal "justice" systems, barroom scuffles, and domestic violence around the world on a daily basis, a powerful moral imperative to preserve life persists. For many world religions, taking human life is the preeminent moral transgression.

Killing, especially the killing of human beings, is an issue that arouses such a visceral response that it is regarded as a primeval sin. For this reason, it is important to examine what is meant by the "right to die." The phrase sounds a bit odd to the Buddhist ear, because dying is generally viewed as an inevitability rather than an entitlement or right. What is being argued is not really the right to die, but the right to choose the circumstances and perhaps the time of one's own death. Ronald P. Hamel goes into a lengthy discussion about the ambiguity and multiple interpretations of the term.[8] Does the term denote the right to refuse treatment, the right not to have one's dying interfered with, the right to be free of unwanted medical procedures, the right to kill oneself without interference from others, the right to have one's life terminated by someone else, or the right to insist that someone else terminate one's life? Careful distinctions between these possible interpretations of the term need to be made, before we can begin a meaningful discussion of the ethical and legal implications.

As Hamel notes, the term raises questions about a human being's autonomy and right to self-determination, and therefore enters the realm of human rights discourse. As the public debate over the Terri Schiavo case demonstrated, the points of disagreement in the debate over end-of-life issues can be seen to reflect larger faultlines in perspectives on human rights, family rights, divine rights, and the rights of government authorities to circumscribe human freedom. It is important to keep these issues and diverse perspectives in mind, since they are reminders of the complexities involved and the dangers of misunderstandings that may result from muddled thinking, oversimplification, or cultural assumptions about the issues.

The arguments advanced in support of the right to choose the circumstances and/or time of one's dying are primarily related to questions of human dignity and quality of life. Proponents contend that human beings have a right to die on their own terms, meaning they have a right to die in comfort with a sense of their own dignity, rather than at the mercy of the medical system.

Decisions about the right to die naturally lead to a consideration of the medical means that are frequently employed to artificially extend the lives of seriously or terminally ill individuals who are in unrelenting and irremediable pain and psychological misery, and lack the ability or resources to maintain adequate personal care. Any one or a combination of these numerous factors might move a person to consider actively or passively seeking an end to life, and the factors involved give rise to many different options and scenarios. To illustrate, there is a vast difference between refusing treatment that would likely be beneficial and not especially burdensome, and refusing treatment that is expensive, painful, stressful, and futile. There is also a difference between "foreseeing" death (knowing that death will likely result from one's action or nonaction and not preventing it) and intending death (knowingly causing death).

In reflecting on these issues and their different possible scenarios, it is useful to further consider some of the distinctions Beauchamp makes. He argues that in classifying and evaluating cases of physician-assisted termination of a patient's life, it is important to assess "the physician's intentions, the causes of impending death, and the methods used to administer death."[9] He further argues that "a value system that puts humanness and personal integrity above biological life and function" may find it "harder morally to justify letting somebody die a slow, ugly, dehumanizing death than it is to justify helping him to escape from such misery."[10]

This line of reasoning sounds sensible and is frequently voiced, but it also oversimplifies some complex questions and masks an underlying set of assumptions about death, human identity, and human integrity. Few observers would dispute the values of human dignity and personal integrity, but it is logically unsound to propose that any code of ethics that values humanness and personal integrity above biological life and function would necessarily sanction taking the life of someone dying a miserable death. There are many world religions with humanistic value systems that esteem human dignity and personal integrity over biological life and function, but would not sanction euthanasia. Buddhists, for example, would not wish anyone to die a slow, ugly, and dehumanizing death, but they would not automatically conclude that euthanasia is the optimum, or the only way to help disabled, debilitated, or dying persons cope with their miserable situations. On the basis of the Four Noble Truths, Buddhists recognize that the sufferings of sickness, old age, and death are normal experiences for human beings and that these conditions, however painful, are neither ugly nor dehumanizing. On the contrary, death is an integral aspect of what it means to be human.

Once the body is no longer able to sustain life, it may be assumed that the person's allotted life span is exhausted. It is impossible to know the state of mind of a person trapped in a body that in no longer functioning normally, but we know from the accounts of stroke victims and paraplegics that immobility and lack of autonomy can be extremely unpleasant and frustrating, so this could be the case with comatose patients as well. At this point, allowing someone's consciousness to leave the body gently and naturally may be more compassionate than artificially preventing the consciousness from transiting to a new state of existence. It would be very useful to develop more accurate ways to assess whether or not a person will pull through. Instead of clinging to the illusion that a person will recover even when the situation is hopeless and subjecting the person to a battery of painful medical treatments, it may be far more compassionate to let the person go.

Buddhist Attitudes Toward Compassionate Killing

Traditionally in Buddhist thought and praxis, the taking of life is regarded as morally wrong, regardless of the circumstances. Buddhist texts consistently state that taking life, particularly human life, is to be avoided, and they include no justifications for circumstances such as self-defense, capital punishment, wars, property defense, or defense of honor. The lack of any exceptions to this nonviolent principle makes the question of taking life, even one's own, relatively unproblematic; all killing is morally unjustifiable. All sentient beings, including animals and other living creatures, have a vested interest in remaining alive, regardless of their physical or mental circumstances. As proof, Buddhist teachers point out that no living being, even the smallest insect, willingly goes to its death.[11]

The Vinaya texts recognize different degrees of severity with respect to taking life. For example, they classify killing a human being as a major transgression (*pārājika*, defeat or root downfall), which is grounds for expulsion from the Saṅgha (monastic order), but they classify killing an animal as a lesser transgression (*pāyantika*, propelling downfall or lapse). While various degrees of severity with regard to the action of killing are recognized, all actions of taking life are regarded as nonvirtuous, including killing in self-defense. Even in the Mahāyāna tradition, where the ethic of compassion for all living beings may be thought to trump the Prātimokṣa precepts of individual liberation, the action of taking life has serious consequences. The *Upāya-kauśalya-nāma Sūtra* story told earlier illustrates this point. Out of compassion, a *bodhisattva* ship captain kills an evil merchant after realizing that he plans to murder the other 499 merchants out of avarice. In this classic example, the *bodhisattva* takes rebirth in a heavenly realm by virtue of his compassionate motivation to save the lives of the five hundred merchants. But before that, he is reborn in a hell realm, though only for an instant, as a result of having killed a human being. The various versions of this story that are told illustrate both the inexorable workings of cause and effect, and also the power of compassion and the importance of the intention that motivates an action.

From a Buddhist perspective, to take the life of a sentient being, whether a human being, an animal, a fetus, or oneself, is regarded as an unwholesome action that gives rise to seriously unpleasant consequences in the future. Because it is an act of taking life, euthanasia is also regarded as unwholesome, even when the sole motivation is to relieve a terminally ill person's suffering. A case of euthanasia documented in the Vinaya tells of a terminally ill monk who is in great pain. His companion monks advocate death, saying that a virtuous person such as he need not fear death. As a result of their advice and urging, the monk stops eating and dies. His companions' actions of praising and advocating death were deemed reprehensible by the Buddha. As a result of this precedent, the actions of praising death, admiring death, and exhorting death are included in the precept against taking life and are likewise regarded as a major transgression (*pārājika*, defeat or root downfall) and grounds for expulsion from the Saṅgha. From this case, which establishes that the actions of taking a human life and encouraging a person to take his or her own life are treated as equally serious, we can conclude that taking a person's life, even at the request of that person, would also be regarded as equally serious.

Keown makes a useful distinction between the immediate intention to do an action and the ultimate motivation behind an action, a difference that is often overlooked in the Buddhist framework.[12] The Buddhists make a useful distinction between immediate benefit and long-range benefit, however. For example, out of compassion, a person may decide to take the life of someone who is suffering from great pain; the action might relieve the immediate pain, but cause far greater sufferings for both persons in future lives. The late Tibetan monk scholar Lama Thubten Yeshe, responding to a question about the possible benefit of euthanizing some puppies infected with distemper, said, "If you know, beyond a shadow of a doubt, that you are creating happiness rather than suffering for these beings by killing them, then go ahead. But who, other than a person with a very high level of spiritual realization, can be completely sure?" From a Buddhist perspective, the ability to see past and future lives is classified as a type of higher knowledge (*abhijñā*) or supernormal faculty that develops as a result of intensive meditation practice and its attainment indicates a fairly high level of spiritual attainment.[13] Without this higher knowledge, it is presumptuous and risky to assume that death is necessarily the most compassionate course of action, even when a person is suffering intensely and irremediably.

In theory at least, a person may still make the decision to take the life of someone who is suffering intensely, based on compassion so great that the person is willing to risk the miserable consequences in order to relieve another's suffering. The consequences of such a seriously nonvirtuous act as killing a human being are said to be hellish, beyond ordinary conception, so, except in the case of a highly realized being acting out of great compassion who is fully aware of the disastrous results of such an action, the decision to take another person's life, even out of compassion, is considered to be misguided in the long run.

Human decision making is often clouded by ignorance and delusion, and decisions are not always motivated by compassion alone. Even with the best of compassionate intentions, one may be risking intolerably painful consequences. In the case of suicide, one may escape one set of painful circumstances in the present, but risk far greater sufferings in the imminent future. In the case of euthanasia, one may be putting a suffering being out of its present misery, but there is no way of knowing what kinds of suffering that being may have to face once this lifetime ends.

Traditionally, there are a number of factors that help to explain why euthanasia is regarded as inadvisable. First, a human rebirth is precious and very difficult to obtain. Second, to take the life of a human being is a seriously nonvirtuous action that results in dreadful future suffering. Third, to terminate the life of a human being prematurely cuts short that being's allotted life span. Fourth, even while experiencing great suffering or anxiety, one can create virtue and gain realizations. Fifth, suffering is the fruition of unwholesome actions created in the past; life is the beneficial opportunity to learn from and offset that negative karma, and therefore should not to be forfeited. Sixth, no matter how great the sufferings of sickness and old age may be, the sufferings of death and future lives may be even worse. Unless a person has lived an exemplary life and is certain that there is no negative karma left to expiate, there are no grounds for assuming that a person will be better off in the next life.

To examine the first reason in more detail, Buddhists believe that human life is precious because: (1) it is rare and difficult to obtain; (2) it is fragile and easily lost; and (3) only human beings have the ability to develop understanding and compassion, progress on the spiritual path, and achieve liberation. A human rebirth is regarded as the ideal opportunity to create merit, develop spiritually, and achieve liberation from *saṃsāra*. In addition, Mahāyāna Buddhists believe that each sentient being (human or nonhuman) possesses Buddha nature, the potential to achieve perfect Buddhahood. Although the goals of the path—liberation, enlightenment, perfect awakening, Buddhahood—may be defined differently in the lexicons of the various Buddhist schools, according to the Mahāyāna schools, all sentient beings have the potential to achieve them. A human rebirth is the perfect opportunity to work at optimizing that potential. Throughout all phases of life, the process of dying, the intermediate state, and all successive rebirths until the achievement of Buddhahood, each sentient being has the potential to manifest awakening or to work toward that goal. To cut a life short, especially a human life, is to forfeit this precious potential. To protect and support life is regarded as worthy because it guards and nurtures this potential. To protect and support human life is regarded as especially worthy, because human beings generally have greater intelligence than other sentient beings and are therefore more likely to actualize their potential for awakening.

As valuable as a human rebirth is, especially the life of a human being striving for enlightenment, no obligation to prolong life is mentioned in the Buddhist texts. The available means of treating diseases at the time of the Buddha were primarily herbs, massage, and health-sustaining foods, and these remedies were sought when appropriate. The artificial means of extending life that are available in some countries today were not available at that time, so we have no way of knowing for certain how the Buddha might have assessed contemporary bioethical debates. On other ethical issues, decision-making responsibility rests with the individual, so lacking references to the contrary, I interpret this to mean that a person is free to choose artificial life support or to refuse it, and must take full responsibility for the decision. A person can take Advance Healthcare Directives into consideration and decide in advance whether or not to request artificial life support, but is under no obligation to extend the dying process by extraordinary means.

From my examination of the debate and the responses of the Buddhist traditions on two core issues of the debate, I conclude that intractable pain does not justify euthanasia and that the principle to protect and nurture life does not necessitate extraordinary medical procedures. Overall, in cases of illness, Buddhists see no reason to refrain from standard medical treatments. In cases of extremely painful conditions, there is also no reason to refrain from taking or administering pain medication, as long as the patient's life is not endangered. It is not always easy to determine what distinguishes a standard medical procedure from an extraordinary one, however, or an appropriate dosage of pain medication from an inappropriate one. For example, a higher dose of narcotic to treat pain may also dampen respiration by anesthetizing the medulla of the lungs, which may adversely affect the patient's breathing and chances of survival. Skilled meditation practitioners and others may wish to also avoid high doses of pain medication to keep the mind clear and not dull the mind's capacity for mindfulness and alertness. By contrast, patients suffering from depression or severe pain may seek an overdose of morphine or another similar medication, so as to exit swiftly and painlessly. The skilled medical practitioner or caregiver would steer a middle course between under-medication and over-medication, and between neglecting treatment and recommending extremely painful, bothersome, or futile medical interventions.

The Buddhist texts do not argue that pain is to be borne nobly, though suffering is recognized as concomitant with the human condition and therefore accepted as an integral part of the human experience. Still, it is entirely possible for pain medications to be judiciously prescribed. With improved pain management and palliative care, especially the advent of hospice care, arguments in favor of euthanasia based on extreme suffering have become less common. Indeed on average, it appears that pain is less of a factor in wishing to end one's life than previously assumed. In the Netherlands, for example, where physician-assisted suicide is legal under certain circumstances, a survey of requests for assisted suicide found that less than 20 percent of cases were precipitated by the wish to end pain. More common reasons were the feeling of being a burden, inability to live independently, and a sense of hopelessness and futility about life. In general, quality of life arguments in support of euthanasia look different from Buddhist points of view, because happiness is not calculated simply in terms of physical and mental comfort. The texts repeatedly emphasize the disadvantages of attachment to pleasure and physical comfort, arguing that most pleasures are ephemeral at best and attachment to them can easily become a source of confusion and misery. Paradoxically, the ultimate happiness of liberation or enlightenment is gained precisely through renouncing worldly pleasure and desire. Since death is unavoidable, and worldly pleasures are fleeting, it is far more worthwhile to use life meaningfully to seek liberation. The joy of achieving this goal is portrayed as greater than all the paltry fleeting pleasures of *saṃsāra*.

In the Abrahamic religious traditions—Judaism, Christianity, and Islam—the view that life is given and taken away by a creator God, a supreme being who holds human destiny in his hands, finds no parallel in Buddhist belief. Death is not viewed as a penance, a defeat, or a reproof. In Buddhist belief, there is no sense of life as sanctified as in Christianity or divine as in the Hindu view. Instead, sentient beings experience birth, existence, and death as a result of causes that they previously created and now they continue to create the causes for future birth, existence, and death. In place of sanctity as an intrinsic quality of life, there is a respect for life, a recognition that life is precious to all sentient beings, and a recognition that no being wishes to suffer. Depriving living creatures of their lives is nonvirtuous because it cuts short their allotted life span and causes them to suffer. Human life is considered particularly precious because of its utility in the liberative endeavor. Depriving human beings of life deprives them of the opportunity to escape from the sufferings of cyclic existence, and it is consequently regarded as the most serious of nonvirtues.

Judging from discussions of death in the Vinaya texts, it is likely that most Buddhists would largely accept Beauchamp's working

definitions for the variations of euthanasia. In view of Buddhist pro-
scriptions against taking life and the emphasis that is placed on personal moral accountability, the first variation, to intentionally cause
the death of a human being by active euthanasia, would clearly be
proscribed. The texts offer no justification of "mercy killing"; instead,
a person who intentionally takes the life of another human being is
deemed to have committed a *parajīka* (root downfall), which entails
expulsion from the order for a monastic. Keown cites a Vinaya case
that makes this clear:

> The *Vinita Vatthu* includes a case of a criminal who has just
> been punished by having his hands and feet cut off. A
> *bhikkhu* asks the man's relatives, "Do you want him to die?
> Then make him drink buttermilk." The relatives follow the
> *bhikkhu*'s recommendation, the man dies, and the *bhikkhu*
> incurs a *parajīka*.[14]

No matter how serious a person's illness, injuries, or suffering, and no
matter how painless the method to be used to terminate life, it is
generally believed that taking the life of a human being is an egre-
giously nonvirtuous act. In another case from the *Vinita Vatthu*, a
bhikkhu gives a potion to an ill friend with the intention to kill him off
and, when his deed is revealed, is judged guilty of a *parajīka*. Aiding
and abetting the taking of a human life is as serious as having committed the murder itself. When euthanasia is voluntary—that is, when
the patient requests or consents to the early termination of life—the
patient, the physician, and any other caregiver involved all accrue the
nonvirtuous karma of taking a human life. When euthanasia is involuntary, only the physician or caregiver who implements the procedure accrues the nonvirtue of taking life. These determinations and
their karmic consequences differ in proportion to the intensity of the
wish to kill, the cruelty of the method used, the status of the persons
involved, and other factors.

From a traditional Buddhist point of view, it is likely that what
is currently termed passive euthanasia would be condoned, for the
reason that it does not entail the intentional taking of life, but simply
allows death to occur naturally. Theoretically at least, there is no cul-
pability in simply allowing death to take its natural course. Intentionally withholding food and water from a seriously ill patient, who
wants them and is unable to obtain them without assistance, is not
specifically mentioned in the texts, but would be deemed reprehensible by Buddhists, since food and water are necessary requirements

for life, and withholding them would cause suffering and death. The Buddha is known to have remonstrated with monks who neglected to care for other monks who were seriously ill and unable to care for themselves. He instituted a rule that required monks to attend to the ill. From records of life at the time of the Buddha, especially in the Vinaya texts, it appears that medical treatment generally consisted of herbal medicines, massage, health-promoting foods, herbal poultices, and the dressing of wounds. Medicines included cow urine, cow dung, herbs, honey, and food stuffs such as meat, fish, eggs, oil, honey, and sugar. Certainly none of the sophisticated pharmaceuticals, medical procedures, and technologies used to prolong life today were available then. The withdrawal of herbal medications and treatments may have had a deleterious effect on the patient, but would not necessarily have had the same life-and-death impact that withdrawing life support does today.

Because a human lifetime is an ideal opportunity for achieving liberation, the practice of euthanasia or assisted suicide is antithetical to Buddhist thinking. Even a life of suffering and hardship is counted as a valuable opportunity for realization and spiritual evolution. Therefore, no matter how well-intentioned, the notion of delivering a merciful death can be regarded as somewhat naïve. Given the virtual necessity of rebirth in the six realms of cyclic existence, there is no way to anticipate whether expediting death will ultimately be beneficial or harmful. For a person who accepts the existence of just one life, euthanasia and assisted suicide may appear rational solutions to pain and despair, or even compassionate and courageous, but for a person who accepts the possibility of past and future lives, the matter is not so simple. According to Buddhist teachings, the way to eliminate suffering is not through suicide, but through the achievement of liberation from birth and death altogether. Nor is the achievement of liberation so simple; it typically requires many lifetimes of practicing ethical conduct (*śīla*), meditation (*samādhi*), and intellectual development or wisdom (*prajñā*). Although death may appear to be an easy escape from one's present afflictions, it is not considered a wise solution in the long-term, for the results of any past actions that are not experienced in this life will have to be experienced in future lifetimes, possibly under far more ominous circumstances. The opportunity to expend or expiate one's karma is to be welcomed rather than wasted.

From a traditional Buddhist perspective, allowing death to take its natural course would not necessarily constitute taking life. This approach accords with Beauchamp's observation: "In the past, physicians, lawyers, and moral philosophers have characteristically construed acts of forgoing treatment as letting die, not as acts of either causing death or killing." From a Buddhist perspective, allowing a person to die in due time and according to her own wishes is not necessarily an unwholesome act; however, withholding or withdrawing treatment could be, depending on the motivation of the physician or caregiver. If the motivation is to allow the dying person to die with peace and dignity, there is no blame; if the motivation is to take the life of the patient, then it is a "fully constituted" nonvirtuous action of taking life. If there is no motivation to hasten death, but the patient dies from neglect, carelessness, or accident, the caregiver's actions may be deemed reprehensible and are considered nonvirtuous, but they may not meet the criterion of a fully constituted action of taking life.

If a physician withdraws nutrition and hydration from a patient who can no longer eat or drink independently, knowing that the patient will probably die, and if the physician's motivation is to terminate the patient's life, this is equivalent to taking life. If a physician withdraws nutrition and hydration from a patient who can no longer eat or drink independently, knowing that the patient will probably die, but acts in response to the patient's wish to die according to a natural timeline and without intending to terminate the patient's life, this is not an action of taking life. Ambiguities are inherent in these situations; for instance, it may be difficult to ascertain whether it is the termination of nutrition and hydration that causes the patient's death or the physical affliction itself.[15] Even if the affliction is assumed to be the primary cause of death, the withholding of nutrition and hydration may be a significant contributing cause. If a physician or caregiver administers a lethal dose of some drug or suffocates a patient with the intention of terminating the patient's life, the action is clearly an act of taking life. If a physician or caregiver fails to administer an essential drug or hydration or nutrition against the patient's wishes with the intention of terminating the patient's life, the action is also clearly an act of taking life. If a physician or caregiver provides a lethal dosage of some drug or some other means for a patient to terminate her own life, in response to the patient's clearly express wishes, the action is arguably as blameworthy as providing a weapon or encouraging suicide, which the Vinaya describes as tantamount to taking life. In physician-assisted suicide, from a Buddhist perspective, both patient and physician are equally culpable in the action of taking a human life.

In earlier times a death caused by disease, accident, or fasting was most likely considered natural, but recent astonishing advances in medical technology have complicated matters. Today if patients are unable to eat, drink, or breathe on their own, they are likely to be given artificial nutrition, hydration, or oxygen through tubes and ventilators. A host of new issues attend these new developments in medical science. Death at home from natural causes relieves medical professionals of their legal and moral responsibility; ironically, however, once a patient is taken to the hospital, it becomes very difficult to die a natural death. Medical professionals tend to be understandably wary of the rampant allegations of malpractice and litigation, and therefore are inclined to err on the side of extending life at any cost. Sophisticated medical procedures may stave off death from natural causes, but they may also create complications that require further medical interventions, in a seemingly endless cycle. The causes of death are becoming increasingly more difficult to determine as nutrition and hydration are administered artificially and a wider range of medical procedures are applied. Death may even be a direct result of the very medical technologies (chemotherapy, invasive surgeries, medications, and so on) that are designed to cure the patient.

Earlier we discussed several incidents of suicide or voluntary active euthanasia (by the monks Vakkali, Godhika, and Channa) that were apparently condoned by the Buddha. Each of these incidents involves a monk who is accomplished in meditation and suffering unbearably from an acute and apparently terminal illness. Although the cases are reported only briefly, it may be inferred that, in the case of an *arhat* (one who has achieved liberation and thereby expiated the last remnants of karma), suicide might be blameless. But the case makes one wonder why a person who had eradicated all mental afflictions would commit an act of suicide. It seems odd that an *arhat*, having eliminated all attachment and aversion, could become so overwhelmed by aversion to pain as to commit suicide. Further, even if the *arhat* has eliminated all delusions, committing suicide sets an unfortunate precedent for monastics and laity alike. It is regarded as axiomatic that all actions give rise to consequences and, further, that the consequences of actions are experienced by the doer and no one else. This raises a question about how the consequences of suicide are experienced by an *arhat* who has already achieved liberation, that is, whether or not the consequences of actions can be experienced by someone who is free from rebirth. In the Theravāda tradition, the *arhat*'s karmic stream is said to cease at the moment of death, like a flame is extinguished when the fuel is exhausted. If this is the case, since the consequences of actions ripen on the doer, then there would be no one to experience the normally serious consequences of the action of suicide. Also, if Vakkali, Godhika, and Channa were not *arhats* beforehand, how could they become *arhats* after having committed the serious transgression of taking their own lives? And why did the Buddha exonerate them? They may have been so skilled in meditation that they were able to maintain perfect concentration and equanimity while committing the action and during the dying process, but if the monks were able to maintain perfect concentration and equanimity while killing themselves, why were they not able to tolerate the extreme suffering of acute illness? These questions remain unresolved, but are important for pondering the mind's trajectory after death.

Intending to Kill

A spirited defense of a human being's right to voluntary euthanasia is offered by David Heyd.[16] He begins by setting out five premises: (1) life has no value in itself; (2) only meaningful life has value; (3) only a living person can invest life with meaning; (4) the "sanctity" of life depends on a voluntary decision of the subject; and (5) the cessation of life is a matter of choice, not of mercy.[17] He clarifies his position by saying, "Life, in itself, is not sacred; that is to say, even if it has some value independently of its meaning or quality, there are other values that in certain circumstances may be thought of as over-riding the value of life. Life is not an absolute value." He argues that there is no general principle for determining the meaning of life; life has meaning only insofar as it has meaning for a particular person. Therefore, we must respect the meaning people give to their lives, even if they themselves judge their lives meaningless and not worth living. He says that the "voluntary element in the concept of a mean-ingful life" requires us to respect a person's will to live or not live. The right to life that is ascribed to human beings means that they also have the right to die, including the right to die by euthanasia or suicide.[18] On this basis, it is argued that, like property rights, the right to life includes the right to relinquish life. Opponents of this view contend that the two necessary conditions for performing euthanasia—intoler-able pain and a free and genuine will to die—can never be satisfied, because a person in intolerable pain is not clearheaded enough to be taken seriously and a person clearheaded enough to make the request must not be in intolerable pain. Heyd regards this inescapable paradox as cruel and false, however, because the decision to request euthanasia can be made during "a lull between repeated attacks of pain."[19] He concludes that refusing a request for death is a violation of a right and that acceding on the grounds of mercy is a violation of human dignity.

In response, many Buddhists would agree that life is not an absolute value; most schools of Buddhism are reluctant to speak in terms of absolutes in general and absolute values in particular. But life in itself does have value, for several reasons. Life is not valued because it is given and taken away by a deity, but rather because it is a basis for the mental cultivation that is necessary for awakening. Without life, mental cultivation is impossible and all considerations of value, meaning, sanctity, and volition are irrelevant. To say that life has value only for living beings is tautological; a lifeless universe or an insentient universe could care less about value and meaning. Sentient life obviously has value only for sentient beings, for without a sentient subject there is no one to appreciate life or to speculate about meaning. It is also reasonable to assert that sentient life is meaningful whether or not a person consciously imbues life with meaning. To live a life that is consciously imbued with meaning is optimum, because meaning helps make life's inconveniences supportable, but it does not follow that a life that has not consciously been imbued with meaning is senseless. Even a life that appears meaningless may have meaning for others without one knowing it.

Against the argument that a person has the right to suicide, a Buddhist might argue that a person should be prevented from committing suicide because the act is committed out of ignorance and delusion. A person commits suicide because of not understanding the value of life, the uncertainties of the next life, and the karmic consequences of suicide. Because Buddhists consider suicide highly unfortunate, both for the person and a wider circle, efforts to prevent suicide can be considered worthwhile. Although there may be no objective standard for determining whether a particular life is meaningful or meaningless, worthwhile or worthless, the Buddhist texts offer an ethical framework as a general measure, with the indicators of a meaningful life roughly analogous to those of a virtuous life. Overall, a life of virtue is held to be meaningful and a life of nonvirtue is held to be less meaningful, but no life is utterly meaningless from a Buddhist perspective, least of all a human life. To judge one's life as meaningless is to be ignorant of one's potential as a human being.

Beauchamp proposes to define killing as "circumstances in which one person *intentionally and unjustifiably* causes the death of another human being."[20] This definition is problematic for Buddhists, first of all, because it implies that there are justifiable circumstances for causing the death of a human being. Aside from that, it is important to make a distinction between intentionally killing someone and letting someone die by failing to intervene; after all, hundreds of thousands of people die everyday, but others are not necessarily morally culpable for not intervening to save them. To refuse food and water to a patient under one's care is unethical, however; and some may say that not to intervene when a patient refuses food and water with the intent

to die is also unethical. Ordinarily Buddhists would not sanction killing a patient, even out of a compassionate desire to relieve the intense
pain. Even in cases of terminal illness when natural causes of death
are already at work, the action of intentionally causing death prematurely would be regarded as an unwholesome action. There are circumstances, though, when letting a person in unbearable pain die naturally,
without applying extraordinary medical procedures, may be the most
compassionate thing to do. Here, as we shall see, it is important to make
a distinction between nutrition and hydration that a patient is able to
eat and swallow, and artificial nutrition and hydration that requires the
use of medically inserted feeding tubes and the like.

Intentions are of primary moral import from a Buddhist perspective, but taking life by accident is also regarded as killing. For example, the accidental death of a patient through a mistake in medical
treatment accrues negative karma, but the negative force of the action
is considered slight in comparison with an intentional act of killing,
since the motivation was presumably to benefit, not to harm. An act
of killing, whether accidental or intentional, gives rise to karmic consequences in accordance with the intention as well as the seriousness
of the action. For this reason, killing with the intention to take life is
a far more serious moral act than killing accidentally. The consequences
of accidentally stepping on an insect, for example, are less serious
than intentionally killing it, and intentionally killing with a mind full
of anger or hatred is most serious of all. The consequences of an action
also depend on the agent of the action. If a person has voluntarily
made a commitment to refrain from a certain action by taking a precept, but transgresses it, the consequences of committing that action
are more serious than for someone who has not taken such a precept.
Both Buddhist monastics and laypeople may take a precept against
taking human life. Fully ordained nuns and monks also take a precept
to refrain from taking the life of an animal, even inadvertently. They
also refrain from knowingly drinking water with insects in it, stepping
on living grass, or cutting down trees in an attempt to reduce the
number of unintentional deaths they cause. As noted earlier, even if
the action is not carried out, the intention to kill is itself unwholesome
and will yield unpleasant karmic consequences. The Buddha's stress
on intentionality adds an important tenor to the debate about intervention and non-intervention in end-of-life care.

Intending to Die

In contemporary ethics discourse, consent from the patient is pivotal
in determining whether an act of withdrawing or withholding treat-

ment is morally justifiable. Self-inflicted death is considered suicide, but an act of voluntary passive euthanasia is not necessarily reprehensible, since the patient's allotted life span is not unnaturally interrupted. Buddhist practitioners and ordinary laypeople, especially in Tibetan, Mongolian, and Chinese Buddhist societies, are keenly interested in empowerments and practices that may extend their lives. Even when special methods to extend life are not employed, care is taken to prevent shortening it. But if a patient reaches the end of life and does not wish to be attached to a barrage of beeping machines that are painfully and repeatedly inserted and reinserted, but instead wishes to sit by a pond and watch the fish swim by, or listen to music in privacy, then Buddhists would not consider that an ethical lapse.

The dilemmas become more complex when a patient is no longer able to participate in the decision-making process. In such cases, decisions about whether to deliver or withhold treatment and whether to administer extraordinary medical procedures must be made by a third party. In Buddhist societies, it is assumed that the family, guardian, or caregiver has the patient's benefit foremost in mind. Because being alive is a rare and precious opportunity to practice Dharma, it is also assumed that life is to be preserved whenever possible. Even when a patient is old, sick, and suffering, it is ordinarily assumed that to live is better than to die, because each moment is an opportunity to create merit and to improve one's prospects for the next life. When people are incapable of creating merit physically, it is still possible to create merit verbally and mentally. Despite physical aches and pains, old age is a time of great value since there are less distractions and more time to practice the Dharma. The Tibetan tradition provides instructions on mental cultivation called *"lojong"* (*blo sbyong*, mind training) that are especially useful for transforming one's thoughts and attitudes during difficult times. The practitioner learns to view all circumstances as opportunities to practice transforming obstacles to the path of Dharma. The pinnacles of practice are to transform self-cherishing and self-grasping. Thoughts of self-cherishing are consciously transformed into thoughts of cherishing others and self-grasping is transformed into the wisdom that directly understands emptiness.[21] These instructions are the heart of Mahāyāna and the foundation for all higher practices.

Edmund D. Pellegrino distinguishes between desire, intention, and motivation, and discusses their function in determining the moral status of euthanasia, assisted suicide, and nonintervention (foregoing or withholding medical treatment).[22] For example, one may have the desire to kill someone without having the motivation to kill and without the intention of handling a weapon, one may have the intention to unsheathe a weapon without the desire or motivation to kill someone, and one may have the intention to unsheathe a weapon with the motivation to kill someone. Desire, intention, and motivation function quite differently in these scenarios. Buddhist texts make parallel distinctions: desires are wishes or aspirations, intentions are accompanied by actions toward an end, and motivations are the underlying motives that explain why an action is done. Buddhists also distinguish between base desires for self-gratification and higher aspirations, such as the aspiration to achieve enlightenment.

The *Abhidharmakośa* distinguishes three types of intentions in relation to body, speech, and mind: (1) the conscious intention that directs bodily movements (*kāyaviññatti*); (2) the conscious intention that directs vocal utterances (*vacīviññatti*); and (3) mental intentions (*cetanā*). In Mahāyāna, mental intention (*cetanā*) is also translated as volition and is regarded as the primary instigator of actions. In Pellegrino's view, "A moral event consists of at least four elements: an action, the circumstances under which it is taken, the consequences of the act, and its intention."[23] In Buddhist ethics, there is also a set of four factors that determine the ethical impact of an action: object, intention, action, and the completion of the action. The object may be a mosquito, the intention is to kill the mosquito, the action is carrying through and killing the mosquito, and the completion of the action is the satisfied thought, "Got it!" or the fulfillment of the intention. The main difference between this and Pellagrino's schema is that the Buddhists do not list separately the circumstances under which an action is taken; the circumstances are factored into the weightiness of the action.

Intentionality is a significant common denominator in Buddhist and European systems of ethics. For Buddhists, as for Thomas Aquinas, the motivation behind an action lends special power to an action, whether constructive or destructive. As for Abelard, good intentions are in themselves virtuous mental actions. In the Buddhist schema, however, there are four factors that determine the consequences of an action. To illustrate, an action of killing has significantly different karmic consequences depending on: (1) the status of the agent (i.e., whether the agent of the action has taken a precept against killing or not); (2) the status of the object (whether the object of the action of killing is a human being or an animal, has taken precepts or not, is ordinary or saintly, and so on); (3) the intention (whether to benefit or to harm); (4) the nature of the action (killing or saving lives, stealing or charity, sexual misconduct or chastity, and so on); (5) the manner of executing the action (whether with malice, compassion, or mindlessly); and (6) the result (whether the action is successfully completed or not). The extent to which these criteria are fulfilled correlates with the gravity of the consequences, though much also depends on the specific situation. The *Vibhanga* states that for an action to be complete, four criteria must be present: object, intention, action, and completion. An example of a complete nonvirtuous action is: (1) a specific human being or animal is identified; (2) the intention to kill is generated; (3) the act of killing is committed; and (4) the person or animal dies. The same four criteria apply in the case of a virtuous action.

The question of intentionality is also not easily reduced to a set formula. To begin with, although the motivation behind an action is highly significant, and good intentions are virtuous in themselves, good intentions alone do not ensure that wholesome actions are carried out, nor do they necessarily mitigate the consequences of unskillful acts. Skillful actions are not all well-intentioned either. Highest on the Buddhist scale of ethics are virtuous deeds done with a pure motivation; lowest are nonvirtuous deeds committed with malice. Beings are morally responsible for actions created out of ignorance (for example, animal sacrifice) or carelessness (for example, killing insects while walking or driving), but the consequences are less serious than actions done knowingly and deliberately. The consequences of an action are mitigated in a case of mistaken identity, for example, killing one's mother by accident when attempting to kill someone else.[24] Pellegrino's argument that killing weakens the intuitive human prohibition against killing is paralleled by the Buddhist theory that killing imprints the mind stream with a predisposition to kill.

The debate about euthanasia becomes even more complex when it concerns the right to terminate the life of a patient who may be in extreme suffering but is not competent to make decisions and has made no prior provisions, such as in a living will or advance healthcare directive, that would empower family members and physicians to withhold or withdraw medical treatment.[25] Two prevalent contending views are: (1) that a patient in these circumstances has a right to be relieved of suffering ("substituted judgment," "best interests," and so on); and (2) that no one has the right to make such decisions. Reasons for the latter view include the "slippery slope" argument—that people will become inured to murder and their moral sensibilities diminished—and also the critical questions of who decides and by what criteria? In emergency rooms across the United States today, if there is no next-of-kin to intervene, all patients who "code" (i.e., their heart stops) must be resuscitated, even someone 110 years old and in the last stages of terminal cancer.[26] The cost of these practices is enormous in terms of finances, stress caused to the family, and the physical and psychological trauma of futile attempts to resuscitate a person who lies dying. The financial costs raise the critical issue of priorities and disparities in the allocation of resources. Each day expensive medical interventions are provided for a small privileged segment of the world's population, while forty thousand children are said to suffer death from starvation. On what grounds can these disparities be justified? Is it justifiable to put starving children out of their misery? Would they willingly agree? How can one be sure that "best interests" decisions are free of biases such as race, class, and gender?

Contemporary discussions of euthanasia usually focus on issues of quality of life and the viability of life, but quality of life may be viewed quite differently in different cultures. Among Buddhists, for example, a quality life is one that is ethical and meaningful, and questions related to the control of bodily functions or the ability to care for oneself are less relevant. The values of respect for elders, caring for one's parents, and compassion for the sick and suffering are so deeply ingrained throughout life that becoming a burden is not such an issue. The ordinary indicators of quality in contemporary Western society may even contradict what is valuable and meaningful for many Buddhists. Youth and old age are not in conflict, since living authentically naturally prepares one for aging and dying. Methods of training the mind prepare one to cope with the realities of old age and death. In seeking to define quality of life and the viability of human life in an increasingly multicultural world, therefore, it is essential to realize that a "good death" is not the same for all.

A Good Buddhist Death

Views about what constitutes a good death and even about when death occurs may differ widely among Buddhist scholars and adherents in different traditions and cultures. At present the prevailing view, among those familiar with the issues, is that as long as the brain stem is functioning, an individual's integrity as a person should be respected. This would include providing nutrition, hydration, and other personal care. Opinions differ on questions about individuals who are in a persistent vegetative state, however. Some feel that the ability to react to outside stimuli indicates that the consciousness may still be present in the body, while others point out that vegetable life often reacts to outside stimuli, even in the absence of consciousness. In Damien Keown's assessment, brain stem death is a reasonable criterion for judging the death of a human person: "Brain stem death means that the patient has lost irreversibly the capacity for integrated organic functioning. Its occurrence means that the capacity for spontaneous respiration has been irretrievably lost, that heartbeat has ceased (or will shortly do so) and that bodily heat will disappear."[27] However, if the heart has not stopped beating and the bodily heat has not yet disappeared, there is reason to believe that the consciousness may still be present in the body. The Thai physician monk Mettananda equates brain stem death with the departure of consciousness, and regards this as the most crucial factor in determining whether death has occurred. Keown, on the other hand, rejects this view as dualistic and prefers to regard the human being as a unitary functioning whole and death as "the death of the whole psycho-physical organism rather than any one of its parts."

Although brain death may signal the departure of consciousness, I believe that it is best to err on the side of caution. As long as there is heat in the body, and a pulse and respiration, or any reflexes, it is best to avoid disturbing the patient, in case the consciousness is present. I disagree with Louis van Loon that brain death denotes cognitive death, because a form of consciousness more subtle than that of cognitive consciousness may operate independently of either gross or subtle brain functions. Even when it has been ascertained that the brain stem is no longer functioning, some would say that a person's integrity should be respected, because the consciousness may still be present in or near the body and should not be disturbed. If the consciousness is still present, it is possible to maintain awareness and achieve realizations. If it is not, nothing has been lost.

Compassionate Care of the Dying

In addition to the physical, emotional, and psychological well-being of the dying, attention is increasingly turning to the spiritual well-being of the terminally ill. Liberating insight into the nature of reality is something that can occur at any time. Not only is spiritual insight as possible for the dying as it is for the living, but it may even be heightened by circumstances of pain and suffering. Suffering is often a catalyst for spiritual growth. This may be especially true in Buddhism, where realizing the suffering nature of cyclic existence is a bona fide spiritual achievement. In place of active or involuntary euthanasia, most Buddhists would probably prefer alternatives such as counseling about death, effective pain management, and compassionate hospice care. In addition, many will recommend Buddhist practices for understanding the inevitability of death and dying, and for mindfully negotiating the dying trajectory. Seasoned Buddhist practitioners view death as a once in a lifetime opportunity for realization and, theoretically at least, enlightenment.

The moment of death is a great opportunity for realization. Coming face-to-face with death and impermanence, suffering, and the immanent dissolution of the illusory self are all opportunities for gaining insight into these basic Buddhist truths. Sufferings can be understood as the result of one's own actions in the past, rather than some inexplicable injustice. Through the experience of suffering of illness and approaching death, this negative karma is expiated and it is possible to achieve profound realizations of suffering, impermanence, karma, and much else. To cut short a life prematurely merely perpetuates the suffering; it simply postpones the suffering to another time, when it might be even more unbearable, and it sows the seeds of further, even greater sufferings through the nonvirtue of taking life.

From a philosophical perspective, it is also possible to reflect on the insubstantial nature of the body and mind at the time of death. Clinging to the body creates tremendous tension that actually increases physical as well as mental pain. Meditation on impermanence relaxes the preconceptions of the mind and expectations of one's own physical continuity, which results in a feeling of greater ease and well-being. Similarly, through meditation on emptiness, an experienced practitioner can dissolve the mental constructs of permanence and solidity that are based on a mistaken understanding of reality. Deconstructing this mistaken view of reality directly challenges the patterns of clinging and grasping at the self, and dispels the sufferings caused by clinging and grasping as death looms near.

There is also a belief that karmic consequences can be purified through spiritual practice. The consequences of a negative deed can be purified in advance through engaging in wholesome deeds to allay the painful consequences of the negative action ripening. It is believed that virtuous actions can offset or outweigh the results of unwholesome actions, just as the effects of a small amount of salt water are neutralized in a huge body of fresh water. Intensive Dharma practice is considered especially effective for purifying the consequences of past nonvirtuous deeds; sometimes the effects are thought to be expiated through enduring a painful illness, for example. For the Buddhists, anxiety about death is not entirely misplaced; in fact, contemplation on death is a healthy motivating factor to spiritual practice, that spurs one to confront the sufferings of life and their source. Satisfaction is not possible in this mortal frame; by resigning oneself to experiencing and understanding the nature of pain and dissatisfaction, one gains knowledge and insight, decreases ignorance, and takes a step forward toward the all-knowing wisdom of a Buddha.

The issues of quality of life, death with dignity, and bodily rights can be approached from very different sets of assumptions about life and death. For example, Buddhists believe that the quality of a life has more to do with character than with bodily functions. A person who has lived a noble life is likely to die a noble death. The crucial issue of human suffering cannot be easily resolved at the last moment, but should be contemplated throughout life, so it does not come as a surprise at the end of life. A quality life is created on the basis of virtuous conduct, generosity, wisdom, and everyday kindness. Life with dignity for Buddhists, then, has less to do with physiology and more to do with psychology.

Meanwhile, we confront such questions as the value of a severely disabled life. From a purely material perspective, a severely disabled life may seem futile and death a desirable alternative. But because life and death are integrally linked with personal meaning and identity, these complex questions deserve to be examined from a variety of perspectives, including the legal, moral, economic, and psychological.

In the North American context, the least controversial approach to the euthanasia debate thus far is to provide better care for the terminally ill. From the Buddha's remonstrations to the uncaring monks, we know that he similarly wished his disciples to extend compassionate care to those suffering from illness, old age, and infirmity. An ethics of compassion may help resolve some of the concerns raised by the euthanasia debate and can also inform certain practical aspects of medical care. For example, to avoid the expense and suffering of protracted litigation, contractual agreements to administer particular substances and treatments can be concluded in advance to ensure the patient's welfare and limit the physician's liability. Although legal adequate safeguards will still be needed to prevent abuses, anticipating moral dilemmas and assigning moral responsibilities in advance will conserve resources for providing optimum health care.[28]

Traditional Buddhist views rest on the assumption that delusions such as desire, aversion, and ignorance cloud human beings' judgments, especially under duress. What we desire is not always what is best for us in the long-term. Because suicide and euthanasia are nonreversible, and have extremely weighty long-range implications, they take on a greater immediacy and urgency than ordinary decisions and therefore deserve more careful consideration. These are the assumptions that underlie Buddhist approaches to death, personal identity, and bioethical issues.

Directing One's Dying in Advance

The prospect of extending life indefinitely by artificial means has caused thoughtful people to question the headlong rush to extend life. Not

only are they questioning the extent to which they wish to extend their
own living and dying, but also the living and dying of their loved ones.
The question itself, even if hypothetical, has become an issue of urgent
concern, as such interventions as breathing machines and feeding tubes
have allowed patients to remain in persistent or permanent vegetative
states for years. The limits of meaningful life and human autonomy
rapidly become apparent in the ICU of American hospitals. Ordinarily,
individuals are responsible for their own decisions and the results of
their decisions; when they lie dying, the equation shifts, because they
are not able to exercise this responsibility effectively. The sight of a
dying parent or child immediately raises critical questions: What are the
limits of the Hippocratic imperative to preserve life? What are the limits
of the Buddhist imperative to refrain from harm? What does it mean to
treat all living beings with compassion?

Buddhists generally speak of human potential rather than human dignity. The closest correlate to human dignity seems to be virtue. A person with dignity is one who lives virtuously, or at least
within the limits of decent human behavior. In the debate about human freedom and determinism, the Buddhists come down decidedly
on the side of freedom to choose one's own course. In Buddhist ethical
terms, human beings act not due to genomes, but rather to causes,
conditions, and ways of thinking and acting that were shaped by actions
in the past. Causes are the propensities or imprints of actions created
in the past and conditions are the circumstances that we find ourselves in. Within these parameters of our own making, human beings
make their own decisions from moment to moment. But, who speaks
for dying people who are no longer capable of making their own
decisions? Who determines how the potential of this human life is to
be best respected?

The Buddhist teachings challenge human beings to be mindful
and pay attention. They explain how moment to moment awareness
is both the best preparation for death and the key to a meaningful life.
Regardless of the philosophical context—and there are several Buddhist variations—mindful awareness dispels the illusion of a concrete
world and an individual's complacent space within it. With alert
mindfulness, cultivated through meditation, it is possible to become
comfortable with a contingent self in a transient world. And though it
can be discomforting to confront our own ephemeral nature, it is well
to reconsider our accustomed patterns and definitions before they are
inevitably shattered by death. Mindfulness practice enables us to be
fully attentive to the present moment, instead of perpetually being
distracted by thoughts of the past and future. The past is gone and

will never come again; the future does not yet exist. The present moment is all we have, but often we miss it, because we are stressed out or thinking about something else. In this way, life passes us by and soon it is all over. By learning to pay attention to the present moment, we can remedy these habitual tendencies and begin to live fully, perhaps for the first time.

A person who lives fully in the moment gains a sense of self-fulfillment and may be more inclined to accept the inevitability of death than those who have not made time for self-reflection. If one has lived a meaningful life and has no regrets, the passage should be easy, whereas those who have many regrets and doubt that their lives have been worthwhile may resist death and cling to life, hoping to wring some last pleasure out of it. A person who sincerely believes that a savior figure will ensure a safe passage to heaven may also experience a smooth transition. This can work both ways, however, for if any doubt arises at the last moment, the person may be thrown into chaos and begin to grasp at life, instead of being able to let go. Although the belief in a savior figure is an anomaly in the Buddhist world, adherents of the Pure Land schools in China, Japan, and Taiwan believe that they will enter the Pure Land of Amitābha Buddha due to their strong faith. Japanese accounts of traveling to a Pure Land by the mercy of Amitābha make it appear as if one enters the Pure Land without relinquishing one's present identity. This is both philosophically and psychologically problematic. Though enlightenment is said to be easily attained in a Pure Land, getting there requires an extremely strong faith in the saving grace of Amitābha. If one's faith falters, clinging to self-identity as it dissolves at the time of death may be the cause of great confusion and despair. Whatever one's religious beliefs may be, because of the psychological stress of losing one's sense of identity at the time of dying, prior reflection on the construct of self is essential.

Reflection on the constructed self is equally as important for those left behind. With the loss of a close loved one, one's heart feels heavy and life seems shattered. Familiar supports are removed and a segment of one's own personal history seems ripped away. Even experienced meditators may have difficulty restoring their balance. Rituals can be helpful in the process of adjusting to the traumas of death and separation. Whether rituals help the dying person or not, they undoubtedly help survivors to recover their equilibrium and to process their grief in constructive ways. Whether it be chanting the name of Amitābha, reciting mantras, silent reflection, or prayers, Buddhists find that such practices are helpful in focusing on the present moment rather than getting sucked into the dramas of hospital, family, funeral, and estate that unfold as soon as death occurs. In this vulnerable state, at the very least, rituals can help get ego out of the way long enough to cope with the loss, generate positive thoughts for the dying, and hopefully gain some direct insight into the nature of life and death.

The Debate Over Dying with Dignity

There is an intuitive understanding that something is awry with life in contemporary privileged societies. The artificiality, excesses, fissures, and hypocrisy of living in a bubble while millions die of poverty and disease are not difficult to see, but few are willing to forego their familiar comforts, and therefore do not look. There is also an intuitive understanding of violence as wrong and kindness as right, but many people lack adequate tools for effecting change and decide to ignore problems that are too big to handle. Buddhism provides a framework for identifying the source of the problem and for effecting a transformation in consciousness. However, to expand our options, we must be willing to venture outside all received ideas about consciousness, personhood, and the nature of the world, and be willing to look inside. To get over the idea of a solid sense of self means rejecting the notion of static identity and all absolutes. It means flying in the face of contemporary society and its glorification of the self.

The Buddhist teachings awaken us to the fact that, in the face of death, most of what we hold dear is utterly worthless. If we are honest about death, there will be plenty of time to prepare by living a meaningful life, so there will be no regrets at the end of life. We begin to recognize patterns of compulsive busyness, addiction to pleasure, and foolish self-absorption that is devoid of any ultimate meaning. By reflecting on death, we begin to recognize that we invest our lives in pursuits that are meaningless when measured by this ultimate yardstick. The moment this realization dawns, we have already begun a radical transformation of consciousness. To reflect on our own death casts legitimate doubts on many of our actions in the past and forces us to reevaluate our priorities. Rather that just depressing us, these doubts can awaken us to the potential for immanent transformation of consciousness. Contemplation of death and impermanence is therefore a great teacher. Even if we only have one minute left to live, that moment is invaluable. This reasoning frames the Buddhist position on euthanasia and lends a sense of immediacy to the question.

Practical Methods of Preparing for Death

In today's culturally diverse global society, an exchange of information about practical tools for coping with the universal experiences of dying, grief, and loss can be unifying and mutually beneficial. In this exchange, some Buddhist practices may appear too foreign or too complex, but methods of overcoming anger and jealousy, cultivating loving kindness and compassion, and achieving inner peace and tranquility may be very useful, because they are practical and have parallels in Western culture. Similarly, mindfulness of breathing (*ānāpānasati*), a pan-Buddhist concentration technique, can feel comfortably nonreligious and is therefore gaining wide acceptance as a relaxation technique. Meditation on the impermanent nature of the body, cultivated through awareness of bodily sensations, is another technique that can be applied with great benefit, to foster an intuitive understanding of change. Gradually, more advanced meditations on death and impermanence can be introduced, for those who are interested.

Another useful category of meditation techniques are those that help one cultivate mindfulness in the present moment and an acceptance and appreciation of things as they are. The contemporary usefulness of these techniques is demonstrated by the popularity of Thich Nhat Hanh's many books on the theme: *Present Moment, Wonderful Moment; Our Appointment With Life: The Buddha's Teaching on Living in the Present; Breathe! You Are Alive*; and *Moment by Moment: The Art and Practice of Mindfulness*. Many medical professionals recognize the importance of learning to accept sickness, old age, and death, but lack practical methods for developing an appreciation of their inevitability and for cultivating moment to moment awareness. Buddhist meditation practices can help fill this important gap.

Another beneficial direction for Buddhist/comparative bioethical dialogue concerns the bio-legal dimensions of dying. For example, what would a Buddhist Advanced Healthcare Directive (AHD) look like and what criteria would be used in creating it? The critical need for spiritual advice on such practical matters requires Buddhist scholars to delve into the intricacies of Buddhist ethical theory and create a new applied ethics that stretches traditional philosophical boundaries. What are the ramifications of a "do not resuscitate" order from Buddhist points of view? What constitutes extraordinary methods of prolonging life? Who makes the decisions about end-of-life care and who safeguards them? Answering these questions will require further research into the scriptural and cultural foundations for the variety of ethical choices Buddhists make. To be meaningful, Buddhist bioethical dialogue must include not only the perspectives of Buddhist scholars and religious specialists, but also those of physicians, nurses, hospice workers, legal experts, psychologists, psychiatrists, caregivers, and terminally ill patients.

Buddhists have broadly opposed the intentional destruction of life. Even in the case of a competent person who is imminently dying, and is prepared and wishes to die, there is a cultural bias against the termination of life. Instead, spiritual support systems to benefit both the terminally ill and their families are favored. According to Damien Keown, the Buddhist opposition to the destruction of life includes intentional killing—by both act and omission—but does not include "the administration of palliative drugs, or the withdrawal of futile or excessively burdensome treatment, which may, as a foreseen side-effect, hasten death."[29] The definition of "futile or excessively burdensome treatment" has yet to be formulated in Buddhist societies.

In Asian societies in general, decisions regarding end-of-life care are very much a product of group process. Whether in a family or monastery, terminally ill patients are cared for by their immediate "kin," often without a great deal of medical intervention. Asian societal structures are rapidly changing, but communications between generations are still far closer than they currently are in most Western societies. In the extended families of Asians, the experiences of youth and aging, health and illness, and birth and death are more likely to be familiar topics of conversation than they are in the nuclear-family cultures of the West where the generations live apart. One positive outcome of frequent intergenerational communication is that old and young tend to accept and discuss illness and disability naturally, with less fear and reticence. Intergenerational social and family structures engender an appreciation for the wisdom and experience of older members and encourage supportive networks of caregiving for the frail and elderly—networks that can allay much of the anxiety that commonly accompanies physical and mental decline. Unfortunately, traditional family structures are beginning to unravel in Asian societies, especially in urban environments, and the resulting changes make it essential to rethink attitudes and revise social services. This rethinking of attitudes and social services is not only timely and important in Asia, but in many other societies as well. Greater understanding about the issues that affect all human beings, such as death and end-of-life care, can help bridge the differences that currently threaten human survival.

Chapter 10

Buddhism and Genetic Engineering

The genetic engineering of living organisms represents one of the most significant, controversial, and potentially dangerous bioethical dilemmas facing human society today. The potential for designing children and creating mixed species, for example, immediately raises a multitude of practical and moral questions—questions about proprietary control over biotechnologies, the minimum constituents of a human organism, and the responsibility of justly regulating scientific research that affects the future of all life. Buddhists take a broad view of these issues. From a Buddhist perspective, the ethics of genetic engineering must take into account the suffering and happiness of innumerable living beings, both now at the present time and on into the unforeseeable future. It must also seek to provide the necessary conditions for the flourishing of human beings and other living creatures and their habitats. The evolution of life as we know it has taken thirteen million years and a single misstep could bring it all to a tragic end. The logic of carefully considering all possible options is abundantly clear.

To understand the Buddhist perspective, it is important to remember that there is not simply one Buddhist point of view but rather a very wide range of them. Second, it is good to remember that the views of Buddhist scholars may vary from those of Buddhists on the street. Third, many contemporary issues are not discussed in the Buddhist texts, since the technologies were not in existence at the time of the Buddha. In the absence of references to these specific issues, everything we can say is merely speculative and an interpolation from cases in the texts and oral traditions of Buddhist cultures that are relevant to the bioethical dilemmas of today, so opinions often vary greatly.

At present, there are no Buddhist policy statements on Buddhist ethics, no policy-making apparatus, no procedural norms, and no consensus even about whether it would be desirable to draw up such statements and norms. There is no central administrative body that links the various Buddhist traditions. Even within the different Buddhist traditions, there is rarely any central administrative headquarters or decision-making body equivalent to the Vatican. Although H. H. the Dalai Lama is perhaps the best-known and most respected Buddhist figure today, he speaks only for Tibetan Buddhists at most. Therefore there are no Buddhist encyclicals, no position papers, and as yet very few scholarly studies to use as references.

This raises a question about who speaks for Buddhism. Considering the wide variety of Buddhist philosophies, practices, traditions, and cultures, it is unlikely that consensus on the nature of conception or the status of the embryo could be reached, especially considering the technical nature of scientific research about these topics, for which exact translations rarely exist. Clearly no one can legitimately speak for the Buddhist tradition as a whole. Here I have tried to fairly report Buddhist views, speaking primarily from a Tibetan Buddhist perspective, though I am American, not Tibetan. My purpose has been simply to begin reflecting on bioethical issues, raise questions, and hopefully initiate a conversation to help inform and facilitate decision making among Buddhists and non-Buddhists, not only at the bedside, but also in public health care. Hopefully this conversation will be long-term and will include scholars and practitioners, as well as voices both within and outside the tradition.[1]

Cloning Sentient Beings

A review of the issues surrounding cloning was prepared by the National Bioethics Advisory Commission after the sheep Dolly was cloned in February 1997.[2] However, the review only took into account religious perspectives from the Jewish, Christian, and Islamic traditions. The assumptions these traditions make about death, creation, consciousness, and personhood are radically different from the assumptions that underlie the Asian religious traditions, which went unheard. This is not unexpected. Although diversity is a priority in some government agencies, it certainly is not in all. Moreover, because the technologies are expensive and complex, millions of people in countries around the world have not yet even heard about them, much less had an opportunity to assess them. The Buddhist traditions themselves have yet to undertake a thorough analysis of the issues involved.

Naturally Buddhist texts have nothing specific to say about cloning—a process that was still fantasy even a few decades ago—so Buddhists are left to theorize about the topic and offer opinions based on their interpretations of personal identity and ethical theory. Consciousness is traditionally conceived by Buddhists to be an individuated stream of conscious events that appears to continue from life to life, even in the absence of a soul or independently existing self. The process of causal continuity occurs in different forms from one lifetime to the next and can be conceptualized as a subtle stream of mental consciousness. Each sentient being has such a mental continuum that is causally produced and, in any given lifetime, exists in association with a body. Human and nonhuman animals take a physical body, whereas gods, demigods, hungry ghosts, and hell beings take forms that are invisible to most human beings. According to the logic of the Buddhist texts, consciousness cannot arise from nothing or from physical matter, but must arise from a previous moment of consciousness. Therefore, when a living creature is cloned, the consciousness of the clone must arise from a previous moment of consciousness, too.

The logical extension of traditional Tibetan thinking on consciousness and rebirth is to consider what accounts for the presence of consciousness when human or animal life is artificially produced. According to traditional Buddhist criteria, each sentient being must have its own individual mental continuum. Within this framework, it is understood that each stream of consciousness is associated with a unique physical form and the other aggregates that are the basis for constituting a sentient being. When creatures are cloned, therefore, each creature must possess its own individual mental continuum in order to be considered sentient life. If it were possible to simply clone the body, the body alone would not fulfill the definition of sentient life. The only alternative would be for multiple cloned creatures, whether human or animal, to share a single consciousness, but that is not possible. Contrary to popular myth, because of different environmental and developmental influences, clones are not identical individuals, even though they have the same genetic blueprint. This seems to be consistent with the Buddhist view that each clone must have its own individual consciousness. If cognitive ability were the criterion for sentient life, then the dilemma would be easier to resolve, but consciousness is not necessarily cognitive. The Buddha made this clear in his description of the six types of consciousness, five of which are nonconceptual sense consciousnesses: seeing, hearing, smelling, tasting, and touching.

To draw meaningful correlations between traditional Buddhist views and modern medical science, it is necessary to define what is meant by conception. For Buddhists traditionally, conception is considered the moment at which sentient life begins, which is the point at which conditions are conducive for the incipient being's conscious continuum to begin life in a new body. The word "conception" therefore simply means re-existence or re-linking, absent such notions as divine purpose, conceptual thought, or fully formed moral or ontological status.

In the traditional Buddhist narrative, each incipient being (*antarabhava*) is attracted by desire when it sees a couple, its future parents, in coitus. Somatic cell nuclear transfer or cloning, by contrast, is an asexual method of reproduction. This means that the traditional Buddhist narrative, in which the incipient being (*gandharva*) takes conception by being attracted to the sexual mating of the parents, may be figurative. Otherwise, it becomes difficult to explain how, when searching for a suitable rebirth, the incipient being is attracted to a petri dish, as in artificially achieved conception and somatic cell nuclear transfer. In reproductive engineering, however, fertilization does occur in a petri dish, even though there are no parents in coitus at that moment. Therefore, either sexual desire is not essential to the process of conception *or* the incipient being must be attracted in some other way to the genetic matter in a petri dish. The only other possibility is that the incipient being is attracted to the zygote at some later stage, for example, as it attaches to the wall of the uterus.

Although an outside observer may dismiss the Buddhist explanation of conception as an anthropologically interesting flight of fantasy, it is important to acknowledge the traditional narrative and to take into account the mechanism of desire that is thought to guide an incipient being's consciousness in taking conception. Given this framework, Buddhist theorists must consider why and how such a being would be attracted to take conception in a laboratory setting, minus the stimulus of sexual desire, rather than being attracted by desire to the sexual act elsewhere. If the consciousness of a newly formed clone is not impelled by the standard image of sexual intercourse and desire, the Buddhists must provide some other explanation of how consciousness enters into the process. One alternative is to consider that it is the desire for rebirth that propels the consciousness to a suitable potential body, and that the imagery of sexual attraction is simply a metaphor symbolizing desire. Another alternative is to conclude that desire is not essential to the process of conception, which challenges the Buddhist explanation of the rebirth process.

The stem cells needed for genetic research are isolated before the cells have a chance to highly differentiate. Cell differentiation (for the development of specific organs and tissues) does not begin until the zygote is implanted and begins to grow in the uterus. The blastocyst that implants is two-layered, consisting of inner cell mass and a thin enclosing layer. Stem cells come from this blastocyst stage. It is assumed that undifferentiated cells are incapable of evolving into a human being unless they are successfully implanted.

From a Buddhist standpoint, conception is defined as the "descent" of the consciousness into a suitable conjunction of sperm and egg, which indicates the time of fertilization. In the case of identical twins, the cells divide into two identical individuals at a point sometime between three and thirteen days after conception. The ingress of two streams of consciousness to the twin zygotes would mean that two incipient beings with different karmic trajectories are simultaneously attracted to the identical genetic material. The mere conjunction of biological tissue at conception is not guaranteed to lead to a fully formed human being, however. The conjoined sperm and egg cannot produce a human fetus unless the zygote finds suitable conditions for growth, that is, until it becomes successfully implanted in the wall of the uterus. Even then, a large percentage of implanted zygotes do not successfully develop into viable fetuses. Using this line of reasoning, a case could be made that the ingress of consciousness is most likely to occur after implantation. Yet another argument could be made that, because consciousness arises through contact between a sensory or mental faculty and its appropriate object, consciousness requires a nervous system in order to function. If this is the case, then the ingress of consciousness is most likely to occur with the emergence of the nervous system, which occurs at a point after the successful implantation of the zygote.

Recent research in mammalian reproduction shows that it takes about ten hours for the sperm to reach the egg in the Fallopian tube. The process of fertilization of the egg by the sperm that produces the zygote takes from twelve to twenty-four hours and an additional period of about twenty-four hours is required for the two nuclei to fuse.[3] If the process of fertilization takes such a long time to complete, then the Buddhists must revise their thinking about the process of conception, which according to the traditional narrative, was thought to occur during coitus. In any case, because the process of fertilization of the egg by the sperm requires an extended period of time from coitus to completion, there should be no objection to emergency contraception, no matter how late one sleeps the next morning. The case of identical twins, which result from the division of cells some days after coitus, raises further problems for Buddhists. Because consciousness is regarded as singular, and can neither be multiplied nor divided, it is necessary to explain how two incipient beings may be attracted simultaneously to the nucleus that subsequently divides, and at a time considerably after coitus at that. To argue that fertilization can occur even without the ingress of consciousness is also problematic, because it leaves unanswered the question of how and when the consciousness enters during the embryonic or pre-embryonic stage. All these questions reveal the complexity of establishing the precise moment of the ingress of consciousness and are questions that are currently outside the purview of science.

The questions that are raised by cloning are especially provocative and challenging because, from a Buddhist perspective the migrating being has no independently existing or fixed identity. A group of medical professionals have attempted to articulate a Zen perspective on cloning. They speculate that people's negative emotional reactions to the issue of cloning are evidence that "cloning, in essence, poses a fatal threat to the idea of a discrete individual identity—a kind of death."[4] Although clones are not identical in fact, the specter that someone can clone us and that our identity may somehow slip beyond our control is understandably threatening. From a Buddhist standpoint, however, the sense of loss we feel is only as strong as our sense of identification with what is regarded as an illusory self. The fear of losing our unique individuality is not as strong when we have less clinging to our personal identity to begin with. If our identification is less intense, then we are able to let go of the psychological control mechanism that resents the thought of an identical clone of ourselves. Both the person and the clone can theoretically maintain individual conventional identities, without risking the loss of something more solid. But this argument rests on the premise that both the parent and the clone have individual streams of consciousness. If the consciousness of the parent and clone necessarily have individuated streams of consciousness, as Buddhist theorists assert, then the two are no more similar than identical twins and therefore maintain their individual conventional identities.

The medical professionals in the article I mentioned earlier write from a Zen perspective, a development of Buddhist ideas that occurred more than a thousand years after Buddha Śākyamuni taught in India, yet their findings confirm two important insights of his teachings. As they explore the different motivations for cloning, they discover that most of them are grounded in attachment, even in the case where someone expresses a wish to clone the Buddha. One of their central conclusions is that an accurate understanding of the concept of no-self is fundamental to formulating a satisfactory Buddhist response to the issue of cloning. Echoing the paradoxes in the *Heart Sūtra* and to Nāgārjuna's fourfold refutation, the writers note that, "To say that the clone is identical to the parent is inaccurate; to say that the clone is totally separate and independent of the parent is also inaccurate."[5] The article ends with the well-known Zen *koan*, "What was your original face before your parents were born?"

To take the question further, it is important to distinguish between therapeutic cloning and reproductive cloning. The responses reported above seem to pertain to the question of reproductive cloning, but the issue of cloning organs and tissue for therapeutic research and application may lead to a different set of responses. If Buddhists are concerned with the welfare of living beings, it seems sensible that most would approve of technologies that could lead to cures for medical problems and the relief of human suffering. The issue of therapeutic cloning is not easily resolved, however, because cell transfer may depend on genetic material gathered from human embryos. The research needed to develop cures for currently incurable medical conditions therefore raises a host of ethical issues that deserve fuller consideration.

Few would argue against the use of genome transfer to cure HIV or cancer, but the use of this technology to alter a person's appearance or enhance physical prowess is highly controversial. The human species as it exists today is the result of three-and-a-half-billion years of natural selection. When we begin to tamper either with plant or animal life through bioengineering, there is no way to predict what the outcomes will be. Today many parents are tempted to design children who are taller and smarter, but the consequences of these endeavors are likely to have unintended consequences. There is no way to ensure that altering human physiology or intelligence artificially will automatically lead to human happiness, in fact, it may lead to unanticipated and unsatisfactory results.

In debating the ethics of stem cell research, it is important to draw a distinction between adult stem cell research and embryonic stem cell research, and experimentation using embryos from *in vitro* fertilization (IVF) clinics and embryos that have been created specifically for research. From a Buddhist perspective, a discussion of the ethics involved in *in vitro* fertilization is fundamental to the debate over embryonic stem cell research, since IVF clinics are the primary source of embryonic stem cells.[6] In the desire to replicate themselves rather than adopt children or accept alternative family structures, thousands of couples are turning to the laboratory to craft a child in their own image. In order to create the conditions for a viable pregnancy, however, a multitude of eggs are fertilized. The surplus fertilized eggs are then stored for some future possible use, but after some time are destroyed or discarded. If each of these eggs holds the potential for human life, then the debate about the ethics of utilizing human embryos needs to begin at the source: the profitable clinics that specialize in assisted reproduction.

The desire for assisted reproductive technologies has given rise to many extremely profitable businesses. These businesses are subject to market forces such as competition, profit, advertising, and novelty, and operate without government controls or supervision by external ethics advisory boards. In an environment where the stakes are higher than ever, it seems extremely risky to leave decisions of genetic health and welfare to the discretion of a market economy. Research by private biotech corporations is not subject to public scrutiny nor is it necessarily reviewed by ethics commissions. Although interventions into the human genome are highly risky, there is as yet no effective control mechanism to ensure that the long-term interests of humanity are primary. Decisions to alter the human genetic code should be subject to careful review and discussion, because these decisions affect the long-term welfare of a virtually infinite number of future sentient beings. Procedures to transfer human genes, such as somatic cell therapy and germline gene transfer, may be justifiable, because they hold the potential to cure or prevent diseases and therefore to reduce suffering. Human gene transfer for the purpose of enhancement is more difficult to justify. The risks of allowing human desires to control genetic research are obvious in an era when more and bigger is often considered better.

The primary Buddhist argument against assisted reproduction is that it produces excess embryos that are likely to be disposed of. *In vitro* fertilization makes use of eggs that are artificially inseminated and implanted in a woman's womb. A number of eggs, perhaps eight, are inseminated and two or more of the healthiest looking ones are selected for implantation in the uterus. The remaining fertilized eggs are generally frozen for future use, in case the implanted egg does not lead to pregnancy. There are currently hundreds of thousands of fertilized eggs that have been frozen and stored for possible future use. After some years, perhaps five, these eggs are discarded or destroyed to make room for others. These fertilized eggs can be regarded simply as organic tissue or they can be regarded as embryos with the potential to develop into a human being. In some circles, they are even regarded as human beings.

Age-old questions about the definition of conception and the beginnings of life are again being raised in debates about whether it is moral to use human embryos for research, and whether there is a moral difference between using embryos that were created for another purpose and embryos that were created especially for this purpose. For Buddhists, the moral status of a human embryo that consciously responds to stimuli seems beyond question. If the fetal heartbeat and brain waves of an embryo are detectable in the fourth week, that would certainly indicate the presence of at least the beginnings of a nervous system and therefore a consciousness to process the neurological impulses. Still, it is difficult to pinpoint the precise moment at which a zygote or embryo becomes an ontologically distinct sentient being, because definitions of life differ from culture to culture. These definitions may therefore be regarded as cultural constructs and, as is well-known, cultural constructs change over time in response to historical and social circumstances. In the Roman Catholic tradition, for example, although the current orthodox position is that life begins at conception, that is, when the soul is infused at the time of fertilization, different views on ensoulment have been put forward at different points in time.[7] In the Buddhist traditions, the moment of conception has traditionally been equated with the moment of fertilization. Biologically, however, the matter seems to be somewhat more complex. In a tradition that values logical reasoning, questions about the beginnings of life must be reevaluated in light of new information.

The crux of the debate about stem cell research is the merit or demerit of destroying embryos. The relative merits of using embryos for research, research that has great potential to prevent or treat life-threatening medical conditions, has also set off a lively debate. From a Buddhist perspective, it is important to trace the source of most of these embryos, namely, the *in vitro* fertilization clinics that intentionally create excess embryos in the first place. If one regards these fertilized eggs as potential human life or even full human beings, then it stands to reason that one should be concerned about creating an excess of fertilized eggs to begin with. If one is concerned about the ethical status of these eggs, then one should object to creating excess fertilized eggs that are destined to be disposed of. On the other hand, if one considers fertilized eggs to be simply organic matter, then one may not feel an ethical responsibility to prevent their destruction. In any case, because thousands of frozen fertilized eggs are going to be discarded or destroyed within a given period of time anyway, some people believe that it is morally acceptable or even preferable to use them for research that will potentially cure diseases and relieve human suffering.

Stem Cell Research and Bioengineering

The arguments for and against human embryonic stem cell research primarily hinge on questions of beneficence and non-maleficence. If the central principle is to avoid harm, then it is difficult to justify causing embryos to die, but because this research may eventually lead to the prevention and treatment of medical conditions that are life-threatening, or cause severe disabilities and suffering, some appeal to a weighing of the disadvantages and advantages, or the risks, costs, and benefits. Although this research holds great potential therapeutic benefit, John C. Fletcher argues against elevating research to the same status as healing and prevention in the goals of medicine. He further cautions against blithely assuming that research on excess embryos from IVF clinics is more moral than research on embryos created specifically for such research—known as the created/discarded debate.[8] Many Buddhists would share these concerns. Competing moral claims cannot be reduced to a simple quantifying and weighing of unverifiable potentials, but must be carefully thought through, giving due attention to all aspects of the questions.

The main focus of Buddhist attention is protecting sentient life and the lives of all sentient beings involved in the procedures must be taken into consideration, regardless of future potential benefits. In May 2005, Dr. Woo Suk Hwang fallaciously reported that he and his colleagues used only unfertilized eggs in their human stem cell research at Seoul National University. If this had been the case, Buddhists would have no problem with this type of research because no human life was taken in the process. The more complicated question is whether human life exists from the moment of fertilization; if so, then many human lives are taken when fertilized human eggs are destroyed in IVF procedures or afterwards. A further question is: If a human individual exists from the moment of fertilization (that is, from the moment the egg and sperm become fused), then how do we explain the fact that so many fertilized eggs fail to implant themselves and reach term? According to Buddhist tradition, each of these fertilized eggs is a sentient being and therefore each of them has consciousness. The fact that some of these sentient beings become implanted and develop into mature human beings, whereas others only live for a matter of hours or days is compatible with Buddhist ideas about cause and effect. For instance, sentient beings' life spans may be short if they have taken the lives of living creatures (including animals or insects) in a past life. This could explain why so many zygotes fail to become implanted and why so many embryos fail to reach term.

What It Means to Be Human

The Buddha did not mention the human genetic code or genetic manipulation, so there are no scriptural grounds for either supporting or opposing these types of research or interventions. In the early Buddhist texts, there is no evidence to support a risks-benefits analysis, such that the possible benefits of an action might outweigh the possible harm. Instead, each action plants the seeds of future events. Time runs in cyclical patterns, with both individual human beings and world systems taking rebirth, existing for some time, and disintegrating. Although all causes are said to have their effects at some future time, the patterns of myriad causes and consequences are not linear or specifically predictable, so there is no way to know for certain whether the benefits will outweigh the risks. This line of thinking underscores the value of a moral imperative broad enough to encompass the welfare of all living beings. This framework of moral reasoning must take into account the well-being of human beings and other living creatures, as well as their habitats, now and into the future.

Geshe Ngawang Dhargyey, a Tibetan monk scholar, used to say that what is unique about human beings is not that they work hard and support their young, because many animals do this much better than we do. Human beings are unique because they have the capacity to make intelligent choices, without being ruled by desire and aversion. As Buddhists reflect on biogenetic research, their thinking will be informed by ancient virtues such as nonharm, wisdom, and compassion, and also by contemporary attitudes such as pluralism, secularism, and science. If stem cell research is undertaken for the benefit of all human beings, regardless of race, class, and gender, it has the potential to benefit countless beings. But if this research benefits only a tiny privileged percentage of the world's population, and is beyond the reach of the vast majority who are poor, or if it harms sentient beings, then the advantages must be weighed against the disadvantages.

This sort of cost-benefit analysis raises questions about who will have the authority to supervise genetic research and whose interests will be served. Unless strict controls are established to protect the common good, human embryo research and other biotechnologies could become the purview of special interests. If the future of biogenetics is controlled by self-appointed powers or the market economy, for example, the situation could easily spin out of control. For this reason, it is necessary to establish a community of scholars, practitioners, and private citizens from all religious and cultural backgrounds to carefully consider the profound ethical implications of these technologies, establish standards, and to create a legal framework that is strongly committed to ensuring the best interests of humanity as a whole, both now and in the future.

Despite the philosophical analyses that have been elaborated over the centuries, ultimately Buddhist perspectives are more pragmatic than theoretical, more concerned with practical solutions to pressing human problems than with abstract hypotheticals. A thread that runs through all these analyses and practical applications is the concept of compassion for the suffering of all sentient beings. For Buddhists therefore, at least in theory, providing a good home for a needy child would be more highly valued than producing a likeness of oneself or continuing one's genealogy. Although genealogical continuity is a concern in some Buddhist cultures, it may stem from cultural and social influences other than Buddhism. The Buddhist goal of eliminating the suffering of all sentient beings is not necessarily utilitarian, however, because it does not regard the happiness of the majority as more significant than the happiness of the minority. Rather, the happiness of sentient beings as a whole is taken into consideration and the welfare of no living being is sacrificed, even in the service of the overall welfare of the whole.

To be truly human means to embody those virtues that are conducive to human meaning and benevolence: patience, compassion, and wisdom. Human beings can certainly be greedy, vicious, and terribly selfish, yet somehow these are traits that are considered to be beneath human dignity. From this, it can be surmised that human survival and evolution depend on cultivating benevolence and avoiding maliciousness. All of these criteria are clearly subjective, to some extent, and that may also be pertinent, for evolution is not simply material. What is truly human is not what can be quantified, but something beyond measure. A case in point might be grasping at fertility or extending life, regardless of humanitarian concerns.

Buddhism, Bioethics, and Public Policy

In a pluralistic, multicultural society, individuals will naturally have different ideas about the nature of the human organism, the natural environment, and the ethical limits of human intervention. Since many different types of people and species are all living together on one planet, it is essential to continually create forums for dialogue on how we can live together harmoniously and with respect for our diverse perspectives and ways of life. For example, in some countries, such as Tibet and Saudi Arabia, a conjoining of religious values and political processes is considered ideal. In other countries, such as the United States and India, it is believed that religion and government should remain separate. Now that ideas about the role of religion in government and the separation of church and state are being challenged around the world, it seems more important than ever to listen to religious voices, especially those of underrepresented segments of society and traditions on the margins.

The question remains as to what role governments should play in regulating biogenetic research activities. The limited sample of Buddhists I have queried feel that the role of religion is not to legislate morality, but simply to provide teachings and counseling to guide moral reasoning on actions and the consequences of actions that can be applied to any given problem. Decisions of ethical significance are made with due consideration given to the specific circumstances, including the nature of the action, the status of the agent, the object of the action, the motivation behind the action, and the likely consequences. Ultimately decision-making power rests with the agent of the action, since it is that person who will reap the fruits of the action. Some situations raise ethical questions that extend beyond this simple formula, however. For instance, the case of medically assisted fertility or *in vitro* fertilization raises questions about the disposition of surplus embryos. Killing is proscribed in Buddhism, yet fertilization technologies produce a surfeit of embryos, some of which must be destroyed to produce a healthy child and to protect the life of the mother. Typically only two embryos are implanted, but these two may divide into four, and the risks of carrying four fetuses to term are usually handled by eliminating those that appear least likely to thrive.

Most informed Buddhists see cross-species mammalian bioengineering as frivolous and filled with potential risks. Already bioengineering in horticulture is causing genetic modifications in neighboring fields for miles around, without giving neighboring growers any opportunity for consent or opposition. Genetic modifications in human beings, although intended to enhance certain physical and mental attributes, may have consequences in future generations that are presently unforeseen and possibly harmful. The implications for human choice and the potential for manipulation need to be carefully considered, as well as the implications for biodiversity and human happiness. In contemporary life, the psychological and social effects of intense competition in academics and athletics are already painfully obvious. Buddhists may question how these achievements and the continually higher expectations they engender affect human psychological and spiritual development. The rampant use of steroids, barbituates, and mood-enhancing drugs comes to mind. Although these spheres of activity may bring short-term benefits, they may also bring problems, because human social and ethical development does not always keep pace with material and technological advances. The trust that human beings put in complex economic systems and medical technologies is often misplaced, not to mention the potential for human error. The very strategies that are designed to ensure human happiness may cause bitter suffering, as when savings accounts are pilfered and defibrillators inserted into human hearts are found to be defective. More importantly, through Buddhist eyes, even the most benign and uncontroversial advances are still worldly achievements that may have little relevance or may even be a diversion when it comes to human beings' greater purpose of awakening.

Suzanne Holland raises two important sets of issues.[9] First, she points out the obvious hypocrisy between regulating publicly funded research, while allowing privately funded research to operate free of most controls, through a policy of self-regulation or voluntary compliance. She points out the discrepancy between disallowing human embryonic stem cell research in publicly funded facilities, yet allowing publicly funded researchers to utilize the results derived from privately funded research. She argues that the double standard that currently exists between public and private research undermines the ethical sensibilities of society in general. The promise of therapies capable of replacing diseased or damaged cells with new, healthy cells also raises issues about just distribution and the allocation of public resources. Although human beings are theoretically free to make their own decisions and exercise their own moral agency, the choices of marginalized people may be circumscribed by factors such as economics, education, and access, which are closely interrelated. Insofar as wealth and education are unevenly available in a society, there is a possibility of neglect and abuse, especially in matters of procreative choice. Not to confront these disparities and correct the structural inequalities that afflict marginalized people raises questions about what may be called an ethics of inaction.

Chapter 11

Bioethics in a Rapidly Changing World

The great mystery of death has engaged the human imagination since the beginning of time, but never before have human beings exerted as much control over their own dying as now. Human beings are perhaps the only mammal with sufficient intelligence to contemplate whether and when it is permissible to take their own lives when death approaches, and they still have not come to any consensus on the matter. Throughout history, the question of whether and when life may defensibly be terminated—whether in war, at birth, *in vitro*, in prison—has been contested from various perspectives and people are often inconsistent, opposing death in one instance and advocating it in another. Now that technologies of living, dying, and biological reproduction have become so complex, the debates are more heated than ever. An intelligent discussion about the issues not only requires expertise in a range of areas and disciplines, but also the mental flexibility and openness to consider alternatives.

The pivotal question, germane to all subsequent discussions, is: "When does life begin and when does it end?" But on this issue, again, there is no consensus. In recent decades, medical science has developed certain criteria to determine when the brain is capable of supporting consciousness and when the fetus can survive outside the womb. Medical science has also developed criteria to determine when the brain is no longer capable of supporting consciousness, though these criteria are not universally accepted. The question of when an embryo or fetus becomes or ceases to be a person remains a matter of widely divergent opinion.

Traditional Buddhist perspectives on taking life and hastening death are fairly straightforward. The first precept, to avoid taking life, provides a reference point from which ethical decisions can be made. Negotiation and understanding are preferred to violence, even in a violent or life-threatening situation, and many Buddhists would prefer to be killed than to kill another human being. Today, however, medical science has raised many challenging questions for which there are as yet no definitive Buddhist answers. Questions about bioengineering and genetic cell transfer open up unfamiliar ethical landscapes that require new interpretations of ancient texts and teachings.

The most basic Buddhist criteria for ethical decision making are the principles of nonharm and compassion, grounded in a set of fundamental assumptions about the world and the role of human beings within it. Although there are many divergent streams of Buddhist thought and practice, all accept some interpretation of the law of cause and effect and rebirth, not of the continuity of a personal identity, but of the momentum of an individual's actions from one lifetime to the next. Because the cycle of rebirth encompasses not only human beings but other forms of sentient life as well, the scope of ethical considerations is broader than from many other perspectives. Extending the scope of reference in this way adds further moral, legal, and economic complexity to an already complicated set of issues.

The challenge for bioethicists today is to provide a foundation for ethical decision making that is clear enough to guide moral thinking, and flexible enough to accommodate the range and complexity of new technologies and the biomedical dilemmas they raise. Traditional Buddhist thinking was based on the ethical injunctions attributed to Buddha Śākyamuni and on the commentaries of learned scholars and practitioners written over a period of more than two millennia. The Buddha's injunction to avoid taking life, especially human life, including the life of a fetus, serves as a fundamental principle for Buddhists around the world even today. His further injunction to refrain from encouraging or abetting the taking of life underscores the fundamental importance of the principle of nonharm. These straightforward injunctions have provided standards for making decisions of such matters as reproductive health and end-of-life care. Even today, individual Buddhists seek the advice of scholars who are knowledgeable about the monastic codes (Vinaya) and other ethical treatises. These codes and treatises are now being reexamined in light of shifting value systems, new medical technologies, and nontraditional lifestyles that make moral choices more complex than in the past.

Time and again, the Buddha modified the original formulation of a precept to reflect a different set of circumstances. For example, the precepts that the Buddha is said to have formulated to regulate the monastic community were revised, sometimes several times, to reflect new situations or variations of misdeeds. This process of evolution of the Vinaya regulations for Buddhist monastics clearly shows that regulations appropriate to one set of circumstances may need to be modified in another. In general, the modifications the Buddha is said to have made applied to infractions, not to serious violations of fundamental moral principles, such as the taking of life. For example, the precept of celibacy was modified several times. First, when a monk was accused of having sex with a woman, the Buddha questioned him, ascertained that an infraction had occurred and prohibited monks henceforth from having sexual intercourse with a woman. As subsequent monks became more creative, he similarly prohibited monks from having sex with a man or an animal, or engaging in oral or anal sex. In these precedent-setting cases, the Buddha appears to have recognized that choices are made amid a complex confluence of causes and conditions, and adaptation of the precepts is needed as circumstances shift and individuals test the boundaries of the regulations.

The Buddha also consistently emphasized that individuals are responsible for the consequences of the decisions they make. The question of making decisions for others who are not competent to make decisions for themselves is not discussed. This is just one of many ethical dilemmas that Buddhists today must confront.

Buddhists are still exploring ways of thinking about bioethics and the questions raised by new medical technologies. Over many centuries, the Buddhist traditions have demonstrated flexibility and resilience in addressing the dilemmas of human existence, as shown by the myriad forms Buddhism has taken in response to different cultural conditions. But today Buddhists in all traditions are facing a host of new questions for which there are no ready solutions. Scholars and teachers find themselves revisiting the texts to find authentic and viable solutions to a multitude of bioethical dilemmas raised by modern life. Buddhist texts and commentaries provide valuable resources for understanding and coping with the certainty of death, but they do not speak about issues like stem cell research or reproductive cloning.

Viewed from the broadest possible perspective of endless sufferings in countless lifetimes in infinite world systems, the highest purpose of life and the aim of Buddhist practice is liberation from the entire cycle of birth and death. Viewed in the microcosm of one human lifetime, the aim is to gain insight into the human condition and to develop the potential that human beings have to create happiness instead of suffering for themselves and those around them. These views are mutually entailing and mutually enriching. The enlightened activities of body, speech, and mind that create happiness for ourselves and others are precisely the actions that minimize harm. These, in turn, are precisely the means of ultimately liberating ourselves from the cycle of *saṃsāra*. As Buddhists reflect more carefully on the issues raised by biotechnologies, they may discover new layers of meaning within the ancient texts and greater wisdom within themselves, by having considered questions of life and death on a deeper level.

Verities and Opinions

Contemporary dialogue on bioethics both challenges and enriches Buddhism. Not only do advances in biomedicine challenge Buddhism to reconsider and clarify its ethical stance on a number of issues, including those related to sickness, aging, and death, but they also enrich Buddhism by contributing up-to-date scientific research on neurophysics and cognitive science. For example, medical science may validate or disprove the Buddhist contention that life begins at conception and ends when the subtle mental continuum leaves the body. New reproductive technologies that nurture new life in a petri dish challenge traditional Buddhist narratives about the process of conception. New end-of-life technologies that can extend human life for decades challenge traditional narratives about the process of dying and rebirth.

New medical technologies have also confirmed certain traditional Buddhist beliefs. For example, recent studies conducted at Harvard, Brown, and elsewhere have empirically verified the psychological and physiological benefits of Buddhist meditation techniques, such as demonstrable improvements in blood pressure, respiration, pulse, and a decreased need for oxygen in experienced meditators. Further research may shed light on Buddhist theories of consciousness, the intermediate state, and rebirth. Even if advancing medical technologies neither confirm nor refute Buddhist theories, the impact of technology on ethical decision making will force Buddhists to reexamine and reformulate Buddhist thinking on some of the most fundamental issues of life and death.

Likewise, Buddhist ideas challenge Western medical science by arguing for a view beyond familiar materialist assumptions about the nature, genesis, and meaning of the human experience. When applied to the universal human experience of dying, in particular, Buddhist categories of consciousness and methods for analyzing the workings of the mind and its common pathologies can provide Western cognitive scientists and psychiatrists with new tools and insights. Although each may be forced to learn the other's language, both systems are capable of recognizing their own limitations and can seek a respectful meeting ground where the dialogue could result in a major advance for the field of thanatology. It is no easy task for an adept in any field to acquire the tools necessary to understand an entirely new discipline and begin the dialogue from the ground up, yet new ground cannot be broken until the deficiencies and limitations of the old systems are recognized. Creating the space for a new exploration of consciousness is vital to an understanding of the process of dying.

Some of the psychological dimensions of dying have already been recognized, but there is still a need to develop new ways to explore the experiences of loneliness, fear, and unhappiness that ordinarily accompany the dying process. The emerging fields of thanatology and palliative care are still in their infancy. Currently, specialists in both fields are actively seeking fresh insights and new directions. Now is an ideal time for exploring different perspectives from diverse sources and evaluating the premises on which these other viewpoints rest.

If traditional ways of dying and being reborn met contemporary human needs and desires, this conversation would not be necessary. But because living beings typically fear death and what may lie beyond death, there is strong public support for efforts to eliminate disease and extend life, even without considering the meaning and quality of life. Not only are people living longer, they are also taking longer to die. Whether or not individuals have the right to suicide when living is no longer pleasant or convenient is one question that is being considered. Whether or not they wish to extend life artificially if it means being debilitated, dependent, and miserable is another. Wealth and social status do not always guarantee happiness during the final years of life; in fact, they may lead to bitter disappointments. Surgical procedures are not always successful and even the best medical care may not be able to prevent painful complications. In some cases, disappointments in human relationships verify the Buddhist teachings that wealth and possessions do not automatically solve the problems of life and death. Despite medical advances and material prosperity, many people are more lonely, isolated, and anxious about death than ever before. The state of consciousness of a person lying comatose for fifteen years can only be imagined.

The Buddhist approach begins with understanding that human beings are not independent and substantial by nature, but fleeting and fragile. Meditation practice allows us to discover and appreciate the momentary nature of the mental and physical continuum and to stop clinging to the illusion of a solid self. As we develop insight into the impermanent nature of things, we let go of unrealistic expectations and are freed from the inevitable disappointments. Instead of trying to find satisfaction in externals, we develop an inner sense of contentment that is not buffeted by successes and losses. Recognizing the momentary nature of sense phenomena, we begin to develop a healthier and more realistic understanding of ourselves and the world.

Medical technologies today help assuage the physical suffering that human beings experience, but are less successful at helping them cope with psychological suffering. Unprecedented numbers of people are anesthetizing themselves with drugs and alcohol, but these measures do not directly address the existential pain of being suspended in a life without meaning. People are looking for reasonable explanations about human existence and the meaning of life. As material prosperity fails to deliver anything more than momentary pleasure, thoughtful people seek to understand their feelings of dissatisfaction and frustration. Many are frustrated with the consumerism, greed, and exploitation that now threaten all life. Human beings have few resources to cope with their own self-obsession, or the fear, violence, and anger that rage uncontrollably around them. Meditation techniques that foster insight into the dilemmas and the frustrations of daily life are the very same techniques that are of value in dealing with the dying.

Western theories about death assume the existence of a body and a soul in relationship, and bioethical thinking reflects these assumptions. Buddhist approaches to death and bioethics begin with a different set of assumptions, including suffering, impermanence, no-self, karma, and rebirth. In Buddhist theories, the person is in the body, but is not to be identified with the body. Contrary to the theory of a body/mind dichotomy, Buddhism sees the five senses—sight, sound, smell, taste, and touch—as integrally linked with mental consciousness. According to Dharmakīrti, direct perception is nonconceptual; however, great mindfulness is required to perceive the brief moment of undistorted awareness that precedes conceptualization. The experience of ordinary unenlightened beings is mediated by concepts and therefore perpetually distorted by desire, aversion, and ignorance. The cultivation of mindfulness and alertness enables a practitioner to experience unimpeded awareness at every moment.

Mental consciousness is greatly varied, yet it is only one mode of perception and not inherently superior to sense consciousness. Based on this analysis, the tendency to separate the body and the mind—physical and mental experiences—is highly oversimplified and mistaken. This faulty division between body and mind makes it difficult for sick and dying people to psychologically come to terms with and integrate their experiences of physical pain, discomfort, and disability.

An impaired sense of integration between body and mind can cause debilitated individuals to conclude that a person's worth is diminished when the body becomes frail. Some explanation of the relationship between the physical and mental components of human experience is needed to enable a person to constructively cope with sickness, old age, and death.

The integration of physical and mental experience is verifiable through direct experience, and meditation practice is a practical means for developing an awareness of this interrelatedness. During meditation, it is possible to develop an awareness of the physical sensations that accompany anger, for example. The Western medical system has many techniques for dealing with the physical elements of a dying individual, but has only just begun to recognize the vital importance of dealing intelligently with an individual's psychological state before and at the time of dying. Mental pain must be viewed as equally worthy of attention as physical pain, and not simply masked with drugs and denial. Because physical well-being and psychological well-being are interdependent, families and medical personnel need to be open to new ways of addressing the psychological aspects of sickness and death. Above all, they must be willing to consider alternative solutions to the existential pain that human beings struggle with on a daily basis, especially at the end of life. To treat psychological pain with drugs may be temporarily useful, but is ultimately futile for addressing the existential questions. The Buddhist understanding of the human being addresses these questions straightforwardly and can be a valuable resource.

Buddhism is just one of a number of alternative worldviews that deserve attention, but because Buddhist texts specifically address the problems of sickness, old age, and death, it is an especially rich source of ideas for discussion. Some methods, such as preparing to die mindfully by reflecting on death and impermanence, are found in all Buddhist traditions. Other methods, such as reflecting on the stages of the dying process and the journey through the *bardo*, are unique to the Tibetan tradition. All of these techniques, even those that may seem bizarre or abstract, provide a wealth of ideas that can inform our understanding of death and help alleviate the sufferings that accompany the human experience of dying. Over the centuries, Buddhism has been adapted to meet the needs of people in new cultural environments, such as China, Japan, Tibet, and Vietnam. Today, Buddhist methods for dealing psychologically with sickness, old age, and death can be adapted to meet the needs of modern times and Western society.

The practical application of Buddhist meditative technologies holds great promise in end-of-life care. To be optimally effective, these practices require dedication, renunciation, and sustained discipline, and only a few people in the contemporary world are interested in the intensive training needed for perfect enlightenment. But even without a huge philosophical shift or a monastic level of commitment, Buddhism can be helpful in dealing with the hassles at the end of life and the realities of death.

In the dialogue between Buddhism and Western science thus far, each side generally elucidates its own views, within its own philosophical framework. Participants discuss common themes, exchange information, and note points of convergence and divergence, raising questions that challenge cherished opinions. But culturally the discussants may still live in very different universes. The Buddhist approach to impermanence is based on a direct confrontation with the reality of death. At the doors of temples and monasteries there are human skeletons or depictions of Yama, the Lord of Death, who is ready to seize living beings at the first opportunity. These archetypes are extremely meaningful to Buddhists in Asia, but may simply appear exotic in the West. Visualizing the dissolution of the aggregates or offering one's limbs and vital organs to demons can also seem bizarre from a scientific materialist perspective, but may prove extremely useful during an organ transplant at the moment of death. To find a respectful meeting ground between these two disparate worldviews is a dialogue that is just beginning, and one which may lead to some very unexpected conclusions.

Personal and Political in Global Perspective

As the aging population increases, new medical technologies raise not only theoretical religious and philosophical dilemmas, but also issues of law, politics, and social and economic justice. On a global level, 100 million Chinese are now over sixty years old and the numbers are increasing by twenty thousand a day. In the United States, health care costs are skyrocketing just as millions enter their senior years and the base of younger wage earners and caregivers is shrinking. Because of the potential for abuse (for example, assisted suicide as a solution to pension deficits) and the possibility of human error, even without malicious intent, these issues must be approached with utmost care. The Chinese government is already formulating a euthanasia policy called Tranquil Death to deal with its aging population.

Profound philosophical and religious differences usually underlie opinions on bioethical issues. However, according to the website of a group called Religious Tolerance, a majority of people in Western societies now favor being able to choose euthanasia: 57 percent in the

United States, 76 percent in Canada, 80 percent in Britain, 81 percent in Australia, and 92 percent in the Netherlands. Despite the ever-increasing costs of prolonging life and death, many Americans still hesitate, or are staunchly opposed to the legalization of assisted suicide. Opponents fear that legalizing assisted suicide could endanger vulnerable populations and eventually lead to the unceremonious killing of the disabled and others deemed worthless or burdensome. Although in a liberal democracy laws are framed to protect the rights of the disabled and other minorities, legal systems cannot possibly reflect the interests of all segments of society and legal protections can be altered by the winds of political change. Legal systems based on assumptions shared by the majority may or may not reflect the interests of minority groups.

Buddhists oppose the deliberate destruction of life, but there is nothing in the teachings to indicate that extraordinary measures must be taken to prolong life, or that these measures cannot be discontinued when a patient's condition is deemed to be hopeless. Most Buddhists oppose suicide, assisted suicide, and euthanasia, but not on the grounds that human beings are created in the image of God, or that life is given and can only be taken away by God. Instead, their opposition is based on the premise that sentient beings possess the potential for awakening, which is rare and not easily achieved. Buddhists recognize suffering as an inevitable part of being human and hope to alleviate it wherever possible, so they are not opposed to palliative care. To relieve pain through judicious medication is compassionate, as long as it does not intentionally cause death. Based on the basic principles of nonviolence and compassion, Buddhists generally oppose euthanasia as an act of taking life, since the well-being of the dying person must be viewed within the larger context of future lives and the law of cause and effect. At the same time, they do not insist that life must be continued by artificial means. If death is inevitable, it is morally justifiable to decline life support and die naturally. Human beings are responsible for making their own ethical choices, including those choices that pertain to life and death. Therefore, if they are to make responsible decisions, they should be informed of the ethical implications of their actions. Consequently, it stands to reason that human beings have the right and the responsibility to make known their wishes concerning end-of-life care, in case they are at some future time unable to make those decisions for themselves. Buddhists I have questioned feel that if the dying person has left instructions that decline artificial life support measures, but these measures have already been initiated by medical personnel, it is morally justifiable for those most closely related to the person to discontinue these measures, since they are against the person's wishes. There is no explicit reference to decision making in cases where human beings are incapable of making decisions for themselves or in cases where the dying person has no advance medical directive.

In my understanding, to possess life is not the main issue for Buddhists. Life is present in peas and carrots, but to take the life of a carrot is not considered nonvirtuous. Nonvirtue is entailed in taking the life of a *sentient* being, a being with consciousness. For Buddhists, therefore, the issue hinges not on whether or not the patient is alive, but whether the patient possesses consciousness. As we have seen, a determination cannot be made on the basis of the coarser levels of consciousness, because if it were, the bodies of unconscious or sleeping people could also be destroyed. To avoid this problem, the presence or absence of the subtle level of consciousness must be determined, since this is the minimal requirement for the continuity of a sentient being's life. If the subtle consciousness is not present, there is no harm in burying, cremating, or extracting organs from the person's body, since it is merely a corpse. However, until the subtle consciousness has left the body, it is risky and potentially damaging to dispose of the body or extract the organs.

The critical point for Buddhists is whether or not the subtle consciousness is still present in or around the body, though this is not easy to determine. If the consciousness is still present, it is best not to disturb the body, because any disturbance may interrupt the person's dying process, arousing afflictive emotions such as attachment, fear, or anger, which can lead to unfortunate migrations. Disturbances such as handling the body, inserting tubes, bathing, and surgical procedures are disturbing to patients even when they are not dying, causing pain and irritation. Procedures such as CPR can be especially traumatic and the high incidence of post-traumatic stress disorders indicates that medical procedures can affect patients even when they are apparently unconscious. Although the motivation in performing CPR and other potentially life-saving procedures may be genuinely benign, from a Tibetan Buddhist perspective, to pound on a dying person's chest in an attempt to resuscitate the heart function at the time of death is probably the worst thing that can be done. In the likelihood that a patient might be revived, CPR may be justified. But in the case of an aged and comatose person whose kidneys and other vital organs are not functioning and whose chances of survival are virtually nil, CPR is unwarranted and may be highly damaging to the dying person's future rebirth prospects. At the critical moment when a dying person needs to remain calm and attentive, the trauma of CPR can destroy any chance for a smooth transition and the anger that may be generated can result in a state of mind that is potentially disastrous. It would be far preferable to allow such a person to die in peace, rather than to attempt extraordinary measures to extend life.

Among Tibetan Buddhists, the primary criterion for determining the sentient quality of life is the presence or absence of the subtle consciousness. Traditionally, there are four ways to determine whether or not the subtle consciousness is present or has left the body. In the first instance, survivors consult a reputable *lama*, or spiritual teacher, who uses esoteric means such as divination and meditative awareness to ascertain whether the consciousness has departed or when it will. In the second instance, a drop of mucus, said to represent the white drop received from one's father at birth, appears at the nostrils. Nurses attending dying patients have reported occasionally observing such a phenomenon. In the third instance, the presence of body heat, especially over the heart, is an indicator that the subtle consciousness is still present in or around the body. Since there were no means of artificial life support at the time it was developed, this criterion applies to the case of a person who has died a natural death. In the fourth instance, the body begins to give off an unpleasant odor—a signal that the body is beginning to decompose and a sure sign that the consciousness has left the body. Once the consciousness has departed, the body is referred to as a corpse and what becomes of it is irrelevant. Whether the body is donated to science, fed to the birds, cremated, or buried can no longer harm the consciousness of the deceased or the deceased's future prospects.

The criteria for determining whether consciousness is still present are apparently unique to the Tibetan tradition; other Buddhist traditions may have other criteria for determining when it is permissible to dispose of the deceased's body. In some cultures, there are standard procedures for washing and dressing the body prior to cremation or burial, and a customary interval before disposing of the corpse. In many cultures, there is a prescribed waiting period, often three days, that is observed before the corpse is dispatched. These customs may indicate that other cultures are similarly sensitive to the possibility that a person's spirit or soul or consciousness may not depart or expire concurrently with the breath and pulse. By law, in California and many European countries, it is permissible to leave a dead body in repose for a short period after clinical death. In many religious traditions, the body is left lying in state for some days and a period of three days is quite common. From a Buddhist perspective, it is preferable to leave the body alone until decomposition sets in, rather than to handle or embalm it. After the body begins to decompose, it may be cremated or buried.

To determine whether it is allowable to unplug a patient on life support is a highly complex issue that deserves thorough consideration and is contingent on many factors. If there is any chance that a person in a persistent vegetative state can be revived and live a meaningful life, of course, that potential should be recognized and respected. But it can be very difficult to predict a person's chances of survival and prospects for living a meaningful life. What constitutes a meaningful life varies considerably from person to person; for example, there are devotees of extreme sports and devotees of spirituality. According to traditional Tibetan Buddhist criteria, the determining factor is whether or not the subtle consciousness is still present and, if so, the person should be protected and cared for like any other human being. The difficulty here is in determining whether the subtle consciousness is present. Ordinary means of assessing the presence or absence of consciousness may be able to measure brain function, but current scientific instruments are still unable to detect or measure the very subtle consciousness that is thought to continue from one life to the next. For this reason, from a Buddhist perspective, current definitions of death that are linked to brain stem function are inadequate to determine the viability of human life. The great matter of life and death therefore requires further research, reflection, and dialogue.

The situation of a patient in a persistent vegetative state is complicated by several factors. First, the term "persistent vegetative state" (PVS) is difficult to define and difficult to distinguish from a permanent vegetative state. Second, the criteria for determining whether a person in a persistent vegetative state is "present" have yet to be established. Third, opinions differ as to whether and when it is morally justified or obligatory to provide life support for a patient in a PVS when the patient has explicitly declined these measures. Fourth, opinions differ as to whether, when life support measures have been initiated and the PVS has continued for years, it is morally defensible to withdraw life support. From a Buddhist perspective, the argument that a person must be able to function as a moral person and to enjoy protection as a living human being is flawed. People do not ordinarily function as moral persons while they are asleep or unconscious, yet their lives are still worthy of protection. The argument that a person must meet certain criteria to gauge their quality of life in order to warrant protection also appears flawed. The traditional Buddhist criteria for assuming the existence of a person (technically, the "basis of designation") are the five aggregates—body, feelings, recognition, karmic formation, and consciousness—and the minimum requirement is the existence of consciousness. Persons are impermanent, contingent, and subject to the law of cause and effect, but their right to continue living is considered axiomatic. The current debate over the "right to life," raised by new medical technologies that extend life artificially are forcing Buddhists to reconsider some traditional assumptions.

Buddhists have only recently begun to reflect on the questions raised by biotechnology, but one question to be considered is the state of mind or level of awareness of the comatose patient. Some comatose patients may be aware of events occurring around them, even though they are not fully conscious. During a particularly harrowing, nearly fatal surgery after a snake bite in Delhi, I had such an experience. Although deeply sedated and apparently unconscious during the surgery, I was aware of the insensitive comments made by the surgical staff, who said they did not expect me to survive. I was not only aware of their words and attitudes, but also aware that I hovered between life and death. In the hospital room after the surgery, I appeared totally unconscious, but through a light blue haze I could see what appeared to be angels at the foot of the bed and I thought I had arrived in a heavenly realm. A few days later, I recovered sufficiently to realize that these angels were kind Indian strangers who had donated blood to help save my life. However, according to specialists, a person who is comatose for more than three months almost always has severe brain damage and, after a year, does not revive.

The accumulation of merit is considered very beneficial for those who are terminally ill, dying, or recently deceased. As a person prepares for death, during the process of dying, in the *bardo* state, and into the next life, the performance of prayers, recitation of the Buddhas' names or mantras, and other meritorious acts are thought to be of great benefit both to the practitioner and the dying person. In the Tibetan Buddhist tradition it is believed that, as long as the subtle consciousness is still present, there is a possibility of directing the dying person's consciousness to a Pure Land or even toward enlightenment. If a person is attached to the body or to this life, reading the Buddha's teachings on death and impermanence can be very valuable. If a person experiences fear when confronted by various apparitions during the intermediate state, hearing passages from such guidebooks as *The Great Liberation by Hearing (The Tibetan Book of the Dead)* can be helpful. Until the subtle consciousness leaves the body, a dying person may still have awareness; therefore the integrity of the person's body and consciousness should be respected. Although they have not been clinically documented, the cases of renowned lamas whose bodies remained warm for days or even weeks after the respiration and heart functions ceased indicate that a dying person's body and consciousness should not be disturbed until it is certain that the subtle consciousness has departed. If further documentation can be gathered to prove the Buddhist belief that the process of dying extends beyond brain death, this discovery will have profound implications not only for psychology in general, but also for bioethics in theory and practice.

Ethical Ideals and Social Realities

Many aspects of the contemporary conversation about death have both profound personal significance and enormous social relevance. One of the most poignant social concerns is the relationship between the costs and benefits of advanced medical technologies. While it is fully understandable that affluent families wish to preserve the lives of their loved ones at any cost, we live in an increasingly interconnected global community and we ignore the interests of other members of that community at our own peril. From a global economic perspective, the ever-increasing expense of biotech research and advanced medical procedures raises questions about the widening gap between rich and poor when it comes to health care options. A few multimillionaires amass and hoard capital that could otherwise be used to feed, educate, and prevent the suffering of billions of human beings. A rights-based philosophy premised on entitlement is inadequate to address the urgent problems that face the majority of the world's population that lacks even rudimentary medical care. Since current economic approaches have not been able to satisfactorily address even the most basic human problems and have only increased economic disparities, it is imperative to investigate alternative approaches. Leaving the urgent questions of life and death in the hands of a market economy makes a consideration of alternative approaches imperative.

Buddhists view death as both a problem and an opportunity. Insights can occur at any moment; even moments of pain, the moments while dying, and the moments between death and new life are opportunities for realization. Buddhist ethical theory presupposes that actions have karmic repercussions, and actions such as abortion, suicide, and euthanasia not only interfere with the life process now, but also interrupt the evolution of consciousness over countless lifetimes in the future. Whether the realms of hell, heavens, and hungry ghosts are metaphorical or actual, they figure prominently in Buddhist metaphysics, and are taken quite seriously by Buddhists. Buddhists in Tibetan cultural areas conceive of the *bardo* in richly imaginative terms and continue to regard the interlude between lifetimes as being a time of hellish, heavenly, and liberative possibilities. To avert disastrous rebirths, Buddhists of all traditions accumulate merit, generate remorse for nonvirtuous deeds, and work to transform unwholesome thoughts and emotions into wholesome ones, especially as death draws near. For Buddhists, the experience of dying holds a wealth of opportunities, including the potential for liberation, and should not to be squandered. The smooth transfer of consciousness to the next stage—how one handles death—is far more important than how long one can avoid it. One is defeated by death only when blinded by it.

Buddhists generally frame bioethical issues in terms of karma and mental development, rather than speaking in terms of rights. Buddhists have not traditionally used the language of rights, but this does not mean that patients, women, and fetuses have no rights. The concept of being endowed with inalienable rights fits organically into a worldview with a supreme being who creates human beings in his own image. It does not fit into a philosophical perspective in which there are no divinely created persons or souls to which rights might adhere. For Buddhists, whether an action is ethical or not is determined by three criteria: the intention behind the action, the nature of the action itself, and the effects of the action. Insofar as all sentient beings have the potential to free themselves from suffering, it can be argued that sentient beings have the right to be free from suffering.

In the Buddhist worldview, the theory of *karma* and rebirth serves as a framework to explain the evolution of consciousness and the material world. Whether or not *karma* and rebirth can be objectively verified, these theories are integral aspects of the framework of values in which Buddhists create meaning and make sense of their world. In this worldview, human beings are the arbitrators of their own actions and their place within the evolutionary process. Rebirth and the workings of karma apply to all sentient beings, regardless of species, gender, ethnicity, education, or economic circumstances, and regardless of whether they accept these theories or not. In this schema, a being's welfare in countless future lifetimes far outweighs the benefits and misfortunes of one brief lifetime. The Mahāyāna tradition also emphasizes that the happiness of countless sentient beings outweighs the happiness of a single individual. All these metaphysical strands are closely interwoven in the Buddhist worldview. As idealistic, impractical, or incredible as they may appear to an outside observer, over the course of many centuries the Buddhist worldview has helped billions of people to deal with difficulties and achieve happiness.

Future research on Buddhism and bioethics will not only need to examine generic Buddhist ethical theory as it applies to general questions of bioethics, but will also need to study the variety of Buddhist philosophical interpretations and the variety of practical applications of those interpretations in Buddhist cultures. It will need to delve into how Buddhist beliefs and practices are influenced by both the beliefs and practices of ancient indigenous elements and by contemporary global culture. Questions about which aspects of Buddhist ethics are universal and which are specific to individuals may be less important than questions about the practical relevance and effectiveness of traditional Buddhist ethical ideals in addressing changing social, economic, and political realities. Buddhists will be challenged to formulate bioethical theories that are simultaneously authentic to traditional values such as nonharm and compassion, sophisticated enough to address critical political and economic realities, and flexible enough to dialogue effectively with those espousing vastly different views. To do so, Buddhists must stretch their thinking beyond the personal, familial, and monastic spheres to address a much larger set of issues, including structural inequalities and the discoveries of science. Buddhists need to nurture a generation of scholars and practitioners capable of mastering both the vast philosophical treasures of the Buddhist traditions and also a vast body of new knowledge. To be an effective resource, these scholars and practitioners must be trained to contemplate, analyze, and envision practical solutions to questions and conflicts unimaginable in the Buddha's day. They must be willing to think at the edges of Buddhist philosophy and ethical theory, and to imagine solutions that stretch beyond traditional assumptions.

Just as Western cultural presuppositions challenge Buddhist ideals and assumptions, the Buddhist approach to living and dying challenges Western assumptions, especially about the existence of an independently existent self. Based on different metaphysical views about death, the self, and the world, Buddhists have developed unique practices to cope with and optimize the experience of dying. Although Buddhist philosophies and practices differ, they agree in principle on the ability of human beings to die consciously and meaningfully. Ideas about *karma* and rebirth are morally significant, because they demonstrate that individuals are both subject to cause and effect and have the capacity for independent thinking and action. Whether the notions of *karma* and rebirth are metaphorical or actual, they reinforce the view that individuals experience the consequences of their actions and, at the same time, have the ability to function autonomously in decision making. Persons are contingent (dependent upon their constituent parts, their environment, and so on) and, simultaneously, exert independent moral agency. These ideas provide a starting point for new directions in bioethical dialogue.

Even though Buddhist ideas and meditation practices deeply question and radically deconstruct ordinary notions of self-identity, they are gaining in popularity. An example is Zen practice, which is designed to cut through essentialist notions of phenomena and experience, particularly the notion of self. Equally popular tantric meditation practices begin with the formula: "All dissolves into emptiness," then construct elaborate visualizations that strip away the practitioner's ordinary identity and replace it with the identity of an enlightened figure, the so-called meditation deity (*yidam*). In Tibetan *chö* practice, the practitioner shatters the illusion of an integral personal identity through a visualized offering of the body as ransom for the liberation of all sentient beings from suffering. Other meditation practices include exchanging self for others, in which one exchanges one's own happiness for the problems of others, and *tonglen* (*gtong len*, the practice of taking and sending), in which one takes on the stress and suffering of others and sends them one's own happiness. These practices are examples of practical meditation techniques for letting go of self-cherishing and cutting through the illusion of self. People of many religious backgrounds have found these practices helpful in their own personal development and in keeping with their own religious beliefs.

Challenges of the Self

In earlier chapters, I have argued that Buddhist models of moral personhood, based on nonharm, beneficence, karma, and rebirth, provide a valid foundation for bioethical decision making. I would like to further argue that Buddhist concepts of the universe and living beings in a constant process of change are compatible with scientific materialist and evolutionary models of the universe. Although Buddhist theories are different from many prevailing worldviews, they provide a framework to explain the nature, genesis, and evolution of both the physical universe and consciousness. The Buddhist theory of personhood, explained in terms of constituent aggregates and activated by the law of cause and effect, does not require the existence of a soul, but it does furnish a semblance of personal continuity for everyday practical purposes and is an adequate foundation for moral judgments. Buddhist theories of mental development offer us tools for achieving psychological well-being, and practical methods for understanding and coping with death that are applicable irrespective of ideology. The aim of dying in a calm state of mind, without remorse or fear, reaches beyond religious affiliations. A wise person prepares for the moment of dying realistically and loses no opportunity for insight on the way.

The qualities of loving kindness, compassion, joy, and equanimity (the four *brahmavihāra*s) can be practiced up to the final moment of death and no tradition has a monopoly on them. These qualities are examples of universal values or common denominators that can inform discussions about all the complex questions of whether or not to die a natural death or to seek artificial means to extend life, regardless of quality.

In this attempt to explore Buddhist moral principles as they apply to bioethical concerns, it has become obvious that end-of-life dilemmas must be approached on a case by case basis and are resolved at the discretion of the parties involved. Nevertheless, in introducing the questions, I have presented a number of angles from which Buddhists can begin thinking differently about these ideas. As scientific inquiry expands, the limits of human knowledge about the workings of consciousness and the process of dying become more clear. At present, however, our knowledge is still very limited, often circumscribed by fixed, mistaken, and distorted beliefs. This comes as no surprise to Buddhists, for whom all the conceptual knowledge of ordinary, unenlightened beings is considered necessarily mistaken and distorted.

The complexities of knowing and acting are compounded with each instance of human interaction, as each participant in the process adds another layer of perceptions distorted by individual interests. In the case of an unresponsive patient, for example, the patient's wishes regarding health care may be variously interpreted by each person involved in the decision-making process. The acknowledgment of human limitations both clarifies and complicates moral decision making, but this acknowledgment is necessary for maintaining open gates of communication and learning.

In general, the two fundamental Buddhist moral principles of nonharm and compassion seem completely compatible. After all, if one acts from a heart of compassion, it is unlikely that one would harm any living creature, at least human creatures. But in the case of end-of-life care, there is a possibility that these two values could pose a potential conflict. Imagine, for example, that your mother or another loved one is suffering from the final stages of cancer. Her condition has been diagnosed as terminal and she has wasted away to a shadow of the robust and energetic figure you treasure. Unfortunately she is allergic to the most effective pain medications and is writhing in agony. Her wonderful life is spent and she sees no point in prolonging the agony of dying, so she pleads with you to give her some medication to terminate the agony. Your heart is torn. You want to relieve the brutal misery she is experiencing, but you do not wish to harm her or end her life. In this instance, your compassion for her suffering stands in stark conflict with your commitment to nonharm and the precept not to kill. This scenario depicts what is not simply a Buddhist dilemma, but a dilemma that people of all backgrounds may face. What the Buddhists bring to this ethical problem is that, in this scenario, the dilemma is not only the conflict between life and death, but also the conflict between compassion and nonharm, or even two levels of compassion. The challenge is not to preserve life in any form, at any cost, but to determine what is the most compassionate and least harmful solution, for the patient, the caregiver, and everyone concerned.

At this juncture, it is important to remember that although Buddhists concur on the same basic principles, they may make different decisions in similar circumstances. Buddhist moral reasoning is based on a set of guidelines spelled out in ancient texts, but not all Buddhists are familiar with them. Further, these guidelines are applied in a vast array of situations and contexts by beings of very different backgrounds who may interpret them in different ways. Reflections on Buddhist principles and their applications in practice are therefore part philosophy, part religion, and part cultural anthropology. This rapidly becomes apparent in conversations with North American Buddhists whose attitudes toward ethical decision making may be influenced as much by American values and cultural assumptions as by Buddhist wisdom. The variety of intellectual traditions and cultural adaptations in approaching ethical questions is both daunting and exciting.

Decisions related to reproductive health, end-of-life, and organ transplantation involve many new technologies and bring to light many moral ambiguities. To address these decisions effectively, Buddhists must revisit, reevaluate, and reinterpret traditional ethical theories with all these new, extenuating circumstances in mind. Traditional Buddhist systems of ethics unequivocally disapprove of taking life, including fetal life, but since the time of the Buddha, the range of options and nuances has expanded. Now Buddhists must conjoin their traditional understandings with the finding of modern science to make distinctions between zygotes, embryos, and fetuses, and to determine when conscious life begins. Dying has become much more complicated and medical science is largely responsible, because it has extended the range of decisions to be made at the end of life. Instead of simply taking herbal medications, reciting texts and prayers, and hoping for the best, human beings may now opt for any number of sophisticated medical techniques designed to prolong life and prevent death. Medical professionals now must decide which tubes to insert or remove and when, which medications to prescribe, and when, in what quantities,

and with what side effects. When these efforts are optimally successful, the patient returns home and continues life as before. When these
efforts fail, the patient either dies swiftly or is faced with another
range of complicated options: a regime of rehabilitation, long-term
nursing care, or any number of alternative procedures aimed at preserving life, restoring functions, or correcting the imbalance and damage caused by earlier medical procedures. Life becomes a dreary series
of stop-and-go medical alternatives, with trips to the doctor or the
hospital, negotiations with family and health professionals, and alternating bouts of hope, frustration, and despair. The tragedy for the
privileged is not that medical methods are unavailable, but that they
do not always yield the desired results. In fact, modern medical technologies can produce cycles of suffering and dissatisfaction similar to
Buddhist descriptions of *saṃsāra*. The new technologies require those
with adequate health insurance to distinguish between treatment options that involve short-term and long-term benefits, greater and lesser
sufferings, and different types of risks.

Frankly, because the Buddhist world encompasses such a wide
spectrum of texts, philosophical perspectives, and interpretations, it
will be difficult to reach consensus on all bioethical issues. With no
central institutional authority to issue an official Buddhist policy statement, and an institutional reluctance to extend (much less enforce)
authority beyond the moral directives indicated in the scriptures, responsibility for analyzing these issues and formulating opinions on
them will no doubt be left to individuals. Individuals may seek advice
from their teachers and gather opinions from a range of spiritual
mentors to clarify Buddhist views on specific situations. Because Buddhist ethical decision making is ultimately a matter of individual responsibility, Buddhist leaders and institutions have traditionally relied
on moral guidelines found in the texts, but gathering reliable information from the texts requires years of study and practice, or access to
the trusted and relatively rare Buddhist scholars who have a depth of
understanding based on years of practice. Increasing literacy makes
informed opinion easier to achieve, but considering the sheer volume
of Buddhist texts available in various languages, there is still a steep
learning curve. The emphasis on intentionality is also helpful, but intentionality is subjective and can itself become a source of moral ambiguity. Ultimately practical decision making is left to the individuals
concerned. The fact that the individual is both the subject and the object
of decisions about life and death makes an understanding of individual
identity and the criteria for moral choices all the more critical. The
explorations of informed scholars, such as H. H. Dalai Lama's *The*

Universe in a Single Atom: The Convergence of Science and Spirituality and *Ethics for the New Millennium,* are therefore valuable resources.

The models of moral personhood that are currently used to explore bioethical issues have their limitations when it comes to addressing the ethical complexities raised by advances in biomedical technology. For example, the scientific materialist model of personhood asserts that a person dies when the brain dies, but leaves unanswered questions about the nature and continuity of consciousness, and is inadequate to address the psychological needs of the dying and the bereaved. Beyond the consequences of legal retribution and social disruption, the presuppositions of scientific materialist framework make it difficult to argue cogently against suicide or euthanasia. The ethical theories of the Abrahamic religions are grounded on assumptions about monotheistic creation, an enduring soul, and a God-directed system of moral retribution. Although religious models seem to be satisfactory for significant numbers of adherents, they also leave many questions unanswered. The existence of a soul is not empirically unverifiable and creation theory is difficult to reconcile with the scientific explanations of the physical world. Typical religious models rest on faith in God and salvation, and the theories they advance to explain the evolution of consciousness and the universe do not satisfy nonbelievers.

Whether scientific, existential, or religious, a viable philosophical frame must include a theory of personhood that is adequate to address bioethical dilemmas, especially those related to death. A workable model of personhood needs to provide a basis for making ethical judgments and psychologically satisfying methods to cope with grief and loss. Perhaps in future discussions other, more satisfactory models of moral personhood and more skillful means to analyze the ethical and psychological problems that relate to death will arise.

Buddhist approaches to end-of-life issues pose a fundamental challenge to the ways that death is approached in contemporary societies. The Buddhist approach rejects fixed notions of self as being the basis of clinging, attachment, and suffering, especially in the face of death. Instead, it sees individuals as mutable, accountable to the law of cause and effect, and responsible both for personal ethical choices and the social good. Because one's own welfare is interrelated with the welfare of others, the Buddhists emphasize equanimity, loving kindness, and compassion as the groundwork for the evolution of consciousness and society. Guided by the twin principles of nonharm and beneficence, human beings have the capacity to free themselves from the bondage of self-interest and can help others to free themselves as well.

Notes

Chapter 1: Introduction

1. *Meno* 18b. Quoted in Mircea Eliade, *Death, Afterlife and Eschatology: From Primitives to Zen: A Thematic Sourcebook of the History of Religions* (New York: Harper & Row, 1967), p. 59.

2. *Fragments* 117, in *The Pre-Socratic Philosophers: A Critical History*, trans. by G. S. Kirk and J. E. Raven (Cambridge: Cambridge University Press, 1957). Quoted in Eliade, "Death, Afterlife and Eschatology," *From Primitives to Zen*, p. 57.

3. Hazel Rose Markus and Shinobu Kitayama, "The Cultural Construction of Self and Emotion: Implications for Social Behavior," in *Emotion and Culture: Empirical Studies of Mutual Influence*, eds. Shinobu Kitayama and Hazel Rose Markus (Washington, DC: American Psychological Association, 1994), p. 94.

Chapter 2: Understanding Death and Impermanence

1. Those who immolated themselves in 1963, following Ven. Thich Quang Duc's example, included the monks Thich Nguyen Huong, Thich Thanh Tue, Thich Tieu Dieu, Thich Quang Huong, Thich Thien My, and the nun Thich Nha Trang. Le Thi Thanh Tuyen (Bhikkhuni Lien Tuong), "Vietnamese Buddhist Nuns in the Twentieth Century," M. Phil. thesis, University of Delhi, 1997.

2. A somewhat more elaborate description of the sky burial ritual is found in John Powers' *Introduction to Tibetan Buddhism* (Ithaca, NY: Snow Lion Publications, 1995), pp. 307–309.

3. *Mahāvagga* I.6. In *Vinaya Texts*, trans. T. W. Rhys-Davids and Hermann Oldenberg (Delhi: Motilal Banarsidass, 1982), p. 95.

4. Susan Murcott, *The First Buddhist Women: Translations and Commentaries on the* Therigatha (Berkeley, CA: Parallax Press, 1991), p. 88.

5. Richard Hayes, Buddha-L (Buddhist Academic Discussion Forum), April 5, 1999.

6. Ibid.

7. Bhadantācariya Buddhaghoṣa, *The Path of Purification (Visuddhimagga),* trans. Bhikkhu Ñyāṇmoli (Colombo: A. Semage, 1964), p. 632.

8. Ibid., pp. 633-34.

9. Ibid., p. 719.

10. Ibid., p. 721.

11. Eva K. Neumaier-Dargyay, "Buddhism," in *Life after Death in World Religions,* ed. Harold Coward (Delhi: Sri Satguru Publications, 1997), p. 92.

Chapter 3: Understanding the Nature of Consciousness

1. For further discussion of Buddhist categories of consciousness, see Lati Rinbochay and Elizabeth Napper, *Mind in Tibetan Buddhism* (Ithaca, NY: Snow Lion Publications, 1980).

2. See Zara Houshmand, Robert B. Livingston, and B. Alan Wallace, *Consciousness at the Crossroads: Conversations with the Dalai Lama on Brain Science and Buddhism* (Ithaca, NY: Snow Lion Publications, 1991).

3. Judy Foreman, "The Medical Benefits of Meditation," *Baltimore Sun,* April 28, 2003.

4. Francis Crick, *The Astonishing Hypothesis: The Scientific Search for the Soul* (New York: Scribner: Maxwell Macmillan International, 1994).

5. The formless realm (*ārūpyadhātu*) is not a physical place, but the abode of beings in the four formless absorptions: (1) infinite space (*ākāśānantyāyatana*); (2) infinite consciousness (*vijñānāntyāyatana*); (3) nothingness (*ākicanyāyatana*); and (4) the peak of cyclic existence (*naivasajñānāyatana*). Vasubandhu, *Abhidharmakośabhāyam,* vol. 2, p. 365–68. According to Jeffrey Hopkins, beings take rebirth in the form and formless realms due to particularly strong powers of concentration, but based on ignorance with respect to the nature of the person. *Meditation of Emptiness* (London: Wisdom Publications, 1983), pp. 277–78.

6. English translations include W. Y. Evans-Wentz, *The Tibetan Book of the Dead* (London: Oxford University Press, 1960); Francesca Fremantle and Chögyam Trungpa, *The Tibetan Book of the Dead* (Berkeley and London: Shambhala, 1975); and Robert A. F. Thurman, trans., *The Tibetan Book of the Dead* (New York: Bantam Books, 1994). See also the DVD narrated by Leonard Cohen titled "The Tibetan Book of the Dead: A Way of Life/The Great Liberation" (Wellspring Productions, 2004).

7. Sigmund Freud, *Civilization and Its Discontents,* trans. James Strachey (New York: W. W. Norton and Co., 1962), p. 13.

8. See, for example, Stephen F. Teiser, *Scripture on the Ten Kings and the Making of Purgatory in Medieval Chinese Buddhism* (Honolulu: University of Hawaii Press, 1994); and Stephen F. Teiser, *Ghost Festivals in Medieval China* (Princeton, NJ: Princeton University Press, 1988).

Chapter 4: Contemplating Self and No-Self

1. Bhikkhu Pesala, ed., *The Debate of King Milinda* (Delhi: Motilal Banarsidass, 1998), p. 183.

2. An alternative translation of *nāma-rūpa* is "mind and matter." For example, Bhikkhu Pesala has, "What is it, Nāgasena, that is reborn?" to which Nāgasena replies, "Mind and matter." *The Debate of King Milinda* (Delhi: Motilal Banarsidass, 1998), p. 13.

3. *The Dhammapada*, trans. Eknath Easwaran (Petaluma, CA: Nilgiri Press, 1985), pp. 116–17.

4. This term is also translated as "nonassociated compositional factors." "Nonassociated" here signifies that items in this category (for example, *karma, dharma,* and *saṃsāra*) are neither material nor mental.

5. *Dīgha Nikāya*, vol. I of *Dialogues of the Buddha*, trans. T. W. Rhys-Davids and C. A. F. Rhys-Davids (London: Pali Text Society, 1899–1921), p. 34.

6. Steven Collins, *Selfless Persons: Imagery and Thought in Theravada Buddhism* (Cambridge: Cambridge University Press, 1982), p. 133.

7. Quoted in ibid., p. 125.

8. Bhikkhu Pesala, ed., *The Debate of King Milinda* (Delhi: Motilal Banarsidass, 1998), p. 4.

9. Jeffrey Hopkins, *Meditation on Emptiness*, p. 432.

10. Ibid., p. 161.

11. Elizabeth Napper, *Dependent-Arising and Emptiness* (Boston: Wisdom Publications, 1989), pp. 185–86.

12. The mistaken sense of a self may also arise in dependence on the six elements: earth, water, fire, wind, space, and consciousness, but the analysis of self in terms of the five aggregates is most common.

13. Here I use the term "true existence" rather than "inherent existence," since the Svātantrika-Madhyamaka school accepts the inherent existence of phenomena but, along with the Prāsaṅgika Madhyamaka, does not accept true existence.

14. Jeffrey Hopkins, *Buddhist Advice for Living and Liberation: Nagarjuna's Precious Garland* (Ithaca, NY: Snow Lion Publications, 1998), p. 97.

15. Ibid., p. 101.

16. Ibid., p. 99.

17. Studies on the Buddhist understanding of *karma* appear in Ronald W. Neufeldt, ed., *Karma and Rebirth: Post Classical Developments* (Albany, NY: State University of New York Press, 1986), pp. 123–230; and Wendy Doniger O'Flaherty, ed., *Karma and Rebirth in Classical Indian Traditions* (Berkeley: University of California, 1980), pp. 137–216.

18. For a concise explanation of this process, see John Powers, *Introduction to Tibetan Buddhism* (Ithaca, N.Y.: Snow Lion Publications, 1995), pp. 246–50.

Chapter 5: Foundations of Buddhist Ethics

1. Bhadantācariya Buddhaghoṣa, *The Path of Purification (Visuddhimagga)*, trans. Bhikkhu Ñyāṇmoli, pp. 248–59. Also see Philip Kapleau, *The Wheel of Life and Death* (New York: Doubleday, 1989), p. 62.

2. Literally, "sharing the body with many," that is, the body as host to eighty families of worms.

3. Buddhaghoṣa, *The Path of Purification*, pp. 185–203.

4. Ibid., p. 247.

5. *Saṃyutta* iii.143 and *Majjima* i.296.

6. *Majjima* i.295.

7. The other four are the ascending wind (associated with speech, strength, activity, and memory), pervasive wind (existing in all parts of the body, providing muscular flexion and extension), fire-accompanying wind (associated with digestion), and the downwards-voiding wind (associated with elimination). Yeshi Donden, *Health through Balance: An Introduction to Tibetan Medicine* (Ithaca, NY: Snow Lion Publications, 1986), pp. 34, 45–46.

8. Janice Dean Willis, *On Knowing Reality: The Tattvārtha Chapter of Asaṅga's Bodhisattvabhūmi* (New York: Columbia University Press, 1986), p. 54.

9. Ibid., p. 55.

10. My translation.

11. These three qualifications of the *bodhisattva* are described by Atiśa in *Lamp for the Path to Enlightenment* (*Bodhipratipa*). See Geshe Sonam Rinchen (trans. and ed. Ruth Sonam), *Atisha's Lamp for the Path to Enlightenment* (Ithaca, NY: Snow Lion Publications, 1997).

12. Further details of this taxonomy from a Tibetan perspective are found in Daniel Cozort and Craig Preston, *Buddhist Philosophy: Losang Gönchok's Short Commentary to Jamyang Shayba's Root Text on Tenets* (Ithaca, NY: Snow Lion Publications, 2003), pp. 168–285.

13. See Liu Ming-Wood, "The Yogācāra and Mādhyamika Interpretations of the Buddha-nature Concept in Chinese Buddhism," *Philosophy East and West* 35, 2 (1985): 171–93.

14. Edward Conze, trans., *The Wisdom Books* (London: George Allen & Unwin, 1958), pp. 33–34.

15. Ming-Wood, "The Yogācāra and Madhyamika Interpretation," p. 164.

16. Vasubhandhu, *Vimsatukā-vijñaptimātrata-siddhi*, p. 31.

17. Ibid., p. 26.

18. Willis, *On Knowing Reality*, p. 23.

19. Paul Williams, *Mahāyāna Buddhism: The Doctrinal Foundations* (London: Routledge and Kegan Paul, 1989), p. 85.

20. Paul J. Griffiths, *On Being Mindless: Buddhist Meditation and the Mind-Body Problem* (La Salle, IL: Open Court, 1986), p. 89.

21. Ibid, p. 88.

22. Ibid., p. 82.

23. Ibid., pp. 85–86.

24. Ibid., pp. 95–96.

Chapter 6: Death and Enlightenment in Tibet

1. B. L. Bansal, *Bön: Its Encounter with Buddhism in Tibet* (Delhi: Eastern Book Linkers, 1994), p. 42.

2. Ibid., p. 183.

3. Geoffrey Samuel, *Civilized Shamans: Buddhism in Tibetan Societies* (Washington DC: Smithsonian Institution Press, 1993), pp. 446–47.

4. Cited by Donald S. Lopez, " 'Lamaism' and the Disappearance of Tibet," in *Constructing Tibetan Culture: Contemporary Perspectives,* ed. Frank J. Korom (Quebec: World Heritage Press, 1997), p. 37.

5. Samuel, *Civilized Shamans,* 1993), p. 187.

6. Ibid., p. 186. Samuel suggests that *la* (soul) and *lha* (deity) are related concepts that may have a common source, but others regard the two concepts as distinct. While there may be some overlap, *la* resembles a personal soul whereas the term *lha* denotes a deity.

7. Ibid., p. 187.

8. Tenzin Wangyal, *Wonders of the Natural Mind: The Essence of Dzogchen in the Native Bön Tradition of Tibet* (Barrytown, NY: Station Hill Press, 1993), p. 187.

9. Herbert V. Guenther, *The Life and Teaching of Nāropa* (Boston and London: Shambhala, 1986), p. 44.

10. B. Alan Wallace, *Tibetan Buddhism from the Ground Up: A Practical Approach to Modern Life* (Boston: Wisdom Publications, 1993).

11. Daniel L. Perdue, *Debate in Tibetan Buddhism* (Ithaca, NY: Snow Lion Publications, 1992), p. 354.

12. The *bardos* are described variously in a number of books: Lama Lodö, *Bardo Teachings: The Way of Death and Rebirth* (San Francisco: KDK Publications, 1982); Lati Rinpochay and Jeffrey Hopkins, *Death, Intermediate State and Rebirth in Tibetan Buddhism* (London: Rider and Company, 1979); Bokar Rinpoche, *Death and the Art of Dying in Tibetan Buddhism* (San Francisco: Clear Point Press, 1993); Chökyi Nyima Rinpoche, *The Bardo Guidebook* (Hong Kong: Rangjung Yeshe, 1991); Sogyal Rinpoche, *The Tibetan Book of Living and Dying* (San Francisco: Harper, 1992); and Padmasambhava, *The Tibetan Book of the Dead,* trans. Robert A. F. Thurman (New York: Bantam Books, 1994). Tsele Natsok Rangdrol speaks of four *bardos*: the natural *bardo* of this life, the painful *bardo* of dying, the luminous *bardo* of the *dharmatā* (wisdom of great bliss), and the karmic *bardo* of becoming. *The Mirror of Mindfulness: The Cycle of the Four Bardos* (Boston: Shambhala, 1989). Thurman reminds us that these Buddhist schemata of enumeration are heuristic devices. *The Tibetan Book of the Dead,* p. 35.

13. Yeshi Donden, *Health Through Balance: An Introduction to Tibetan Medicine* (Ithaca, NY: Snow Lion Publications, 1986), pp. 99–101, 104–105.

14. Ibid., p. 18.

15. Thurman, *The Tibetan Book of the Dead,* p. 23.

16. Ibid.

17. Glenn H. Mullin, trans. and ed., *Living in the Face of Death: The Tibetan Tradition* (Ithaca, NY: Snow Lion Publications, 1998), p. 175.

18. Ibid., p. 177.

19. Ibid., pp. 181–87.

20. Padmasambhava, *Natural Liberation: Padmasambhava's Teachings on the Six Bardos,* trans. B. Alan Wallace (Boston: Wisdom Publications, 1998), pp. 196–97.

21. June Campbell, *Traveller in Space: In Search of Female Identity in Tibetan Buddhism* (New York: George Braziller, 1996), p. 209.

22. Janet Gyatso, "The Gcod Tradition," in *Soundings in Tibetan Civilization*, ed. Barbara Nimmri Aziz and Matthew Kapstein (New Delhi: Manohar, 1985), p. 325.

23. John Powers, *Introduction to Tibetan Buddhism*, pp. 370–74.

24. Ibid., p. 371.

25. Ibid., p. 374.

26. William Stablein, "Medical Soteriology of Karma in Buddhist Tantra," in *Karma and Rebirth in Classical Indian Traditions*, ed. Wendy Doniger O'Flaherty (Berkeley, CA: University of California Press, 1980), pp. 213–16.

27. Ibid., p. 106.

28. Ibid., p. 98.

29. Shotaro Iida, "The Nature of Saṃvṛti and the Relationship of Paramārtha to It in Svātantrika-Mādhyamika," in *The Problem of Two Truths in Buddhism and Vedānta*, ed. Mervyn Sprung (Dordrecht: D. Reidel Publishing Company, 1973), p. 67.

30. Geshe Acharya Thubten Loden, *The Fundamental Potential for Enlightenment* (Melbourne: Tushita Publications, 1996), pp. 117–46, 259–71.

31. Sparham, trans., *Ocean of Eloquence* (Albany, NY: State University of New York Press, 1993), p. 6.

32. Ibid., p. 7.

33. Ibid., p. 21.

Chapter 7: The Transition Between Life and Death

1. Arindam Chakrabarti, "Death in Classical Indian Thought," in *Sofies Welt: Ein interreligioser Dialog uber Geschichte, Philosophie, und Wirklichkeit* (Loccum: Evangelische Academie, 1998).

2. Ibid., pp. 13–18.

3. Alex Wayman, "The Intermediate-state Dispute in Buddhism," in *Buddhist Studies in Honour of I. B. Horner*, ed. L. Cousins, A. Kunst, and K. R. Norman (Dordrecht, Holland: D. Reidel Publishing Company, 1974), p. 227. The arguments Wayman gives to support his theory that Nāgārjuna rejected the existence of an intermediate state (pp. 228–29) are not convincing.

4. James P. McDermott, "Karma and Rebirth in Early Buddhism," in *Karma and Rebirth in Classical Indian Traditions*, ed. Wendy Doniger O'Flaherty (Delhi: Motilal Banarsidass, 1999), p. 169.

5. Ibid., p. 170.

6. Ibid. Also see Peter Harvey, *The Selfless Mind: Personality, Consciousness, and Nirvāṇa in Early Buddhism* (Surrey, UK: Curzon Press, 1995), p. 98.

7. Ibid., p. 102.

8. Ibid.

9. Bruce Matthews, "Post-Classical Developments in the Concepts of Karma and Rebirth in Theravāda Buddhism," in *Karma and Rebirth: Post Classical Developments*, ed. Ronald W. Neufeldt (Albany, NY: State University of New York Press, 1986), p. 128.

10. Harvey, *The Selfless Mind*, p. 107.

11. Vasubandhu, *Abhidharmakośabhāṣyam*, trans. Louis de La Vallée and Leo M. Pruden, vol. 2 (Berkeley, CA: Asian Humanities Press, 1988).

12. As a hell being (*naraka*), animal (*tiryagyoni*), *preta* (hungry ghost), heavenly being (*deva*), human (*manuya*), *karmabhava*), and *antarābhava*. Ibid., p. 386.

13. This term is used synonymously with *antarābhava*. It denotes the being that descends to conception in a healthy woman's womb and is sometimes translated as "incipient being." Pischel has "embryo," which is not accurate since the being has not yet taken a physical body. Harvey compares the *gandharva* to a kind of spirit, because it: (1) is subtle; (2) is the carry-over from a dead person; (3) feeds on odors; (4) moves through the air; (5) is similar to the wind (*vāta*); and (6) is parallel to discernment (*viññāṇaṃ*). Harvey, *The Selfless Mind*, p. 106.

14. E.g., *Majjhima* ii.156 and i.265.

15. In the *Abhidharmakośabhāṣyam*, Vasubandhu lists five types of *anāgāmins*: those who attain *nirvāṇa*: (1) in an intermediate existence, (2) immediately upon rebirth, (3) without effort, (4) by means of effort, and (5) by going higher. Although the text is not explicit, the last category may refer to one who achieves *nirvāṇa* in a formless realm (*ārūpyadhātu*), without having died. Op. cit., pp. 386–87. In the *Śrāvakabhūmi*, Asaṅga lists three types of *antarāparinirvāyin*, namely, those who attain *nirvāṇa* (1) at the very moment of accomplishing the *bardo* after death; (2) just after accomplishing the *bardo*; and (3) having accomplished the *bardo* and while heading for rebirth. Wayman, "The Intermediate-state Dispute," pp. 235–36.

16. The five heinously nonvirtuous actions are: (1) matricide; (2) patricide; (3) killing an *arhat*; (4) intentionally causing blood to flow from a *tathāgata*; and (5) causing a schism in the Saṅgha.

17. Vasubandhu, *Abhidharmakośabhāṣyam*, pp. 388–89.

18. The *pūrvakālabhava* is the existence from conception to death. Ibid., pp. 390–91.

19. Ibid., p. 389.

20. Herbert Benson, Robert A. F. Thurman, Howard E. Gardner, Daniel Goleman, eds., *MindScience: An East-West Dialogue* (Boston: Wisdom Publications, 1991), p. 17.

21. These included the Vibhajyavādina, Mahāsaghikas, and the Dharmaguptakas; the dissenters were the Sarvāstivādin Vaibhāṣikas. See Harvey, *The Selfless Mind*, pp. 174–75.

22. Ibid., p. 175.

23. See Margaret Coberly, "Transpersonal Dimensions in Hospice Care and Education: Applications of Tibetan Buddhist Psychology" (PhD diss., University of Hawai'i, 1997), pp. 76–80; Glenn Mullin, *Living in the Face of Death*, pp. 54–58. These reflections are consistent with the eight recollections on death included in Buddhagosha's *Visuddhimagga*, discussed in an earlier chapter.

24. See Coberly, "Transpersonal Dimensions," pp. 80–87, 94–98; and Rinpochay and Hopkins, *Death, Intermediate State and Rebirth*, pp. 32–48.

25. Commentaries such as Tsongkhapa's *Great Exposition of the Stages of the Path* (*Lam rim chen mo*) and Yangchen Gawa'i Lodrö's *Lamp Thoroughly Illuminating the Presentation of the Three Basic Bodies: Death, Intermediate State and Rebirth* (*gZhi'i sku gsum gyi rnam gzhag rab gsal sgron me*), and tantric texts such as Nāgabodhi's *Ordered Stages of the Means of Achieving Guhyasamaja* (*Samājasādhana-vyavasthāli*) describe the dissolution of the mental and physical elements during the dying process.

26. Karma Lekshe Tsomo, "Organ Donation: Opportunity or Obstacle?" in *Tricycle* 11:4 (Summer 1993): 30–35.

27. For a more detailed account of the stages of death, see Geshey Ngawang Dhargyey, *Tibetan Tradition of Mental Development* (Dharamsala: Library of Tibetan Works and Archives, 1974), pp. 24–25; Lodö, *Bardo Teachings: The Way of Death and Rebirth* (San Francisco: KDK Publications, 1982), pp. 1–18; Powers, *Introduction to Tibetan Buddhism*, pp. 287–306; Rinbochay and Hopkins, *Death, Intermediate State and Rebirth*, pp. 29–48; and Thurman, *The Tibetan Book of the Dead*, pp. 41–45.

28. As of this writing, the recent Je Khenpo, Buddhist patriarch of Bhutan, has been is such a state for more than four years. His body is shrinking, but shows no signs of decomposition.

29. Personal communication, October 24, 1998.

30. Bryan J. Cuevas, "Speculations on the Development of the Intermediate-State Doctrine in Tibet." Monograph presented at the XIIth Conference of the International Association of Buddhist Studies, Lausanne, August, 1999, pp. 2–6.

31. Vasubhandu, *Abhidharmakośabhāṣyam*, vol. 2, pp. 386, 500n.

32. Ibid., pp. 386, 507n.

33. Ibid., pp. 387, 507n.

34. Powers, *Introduction to Tibetan Buddhism*, p. 289.

35. Padmasambhava, *Natural Liberation*, pp. 149–50.

36. The term "deity" is a misnomer. The meditational deities (*yidam*) visualized in these practices are not denizens of the god realms, but fully enlightened beings such as Amitābha, Ratnasambhava, Hayagrīva, Vajrapāni, and Yamantaka, or *bodhisattvas* visualized as enlightened beings.

37. *Zab chos zhi khro dgongs pa rang grol las rdzogs rim bar do drug gi khrid yig*. Translated by B. Alan Wallace, with commentary by Gyatrul Rinpoche, in *Natural Liberation*, pp. 81–273.

38. See Padmasambhava, *Natural Liberation*, pp. 3–51; Dhargyey, *Tibetan Tradition of Mental Development*, pp. 39–97.

39. Legs crossed, hands in the lap, spine straight, shoulders level, chin tucked in, lips gently shut, tongue against the upper palate, and eyes gently shut.

40. Padmasambhava, *Natural Liberation*, pp. 103, 207.

41. Ibid., p. 124.

42. Ibid., p. 126.

43. Lying on one's right side, with the right hand placed under the right side of one's head and the left hand placed on the left thigh. This posture is said to facilitate the transfer of consciousness to a Pure Land at the time of death.

44. Padmasambhava, *Natural Liberation*, p. 164.
45. Francisco J. Varela, *Sleeping, Dreaming, and Dying: An Exploration of Consciousness with the Dalai Lama* (Boston: Wisdom Publications, 1997), pp. 122–30.
46. Jeffrey Hopkins, "A Tibetan Perspective on the Nature of Spiritual Experience," in *Paths to Liberation: The Mārga and its Transformations in Buddhist Thought*, ed. Robert E. Buswell, Jr., and Robert M. Gimello (Honolulu: University of Hawaii Press, 1992), p. 244.
47. Padmasambhava, *Natural Liberation*, p. 168.
48. Ibid., p. 172.
49. Paul Williams, *Mahāyāna Buddhism: The Doctrinal Foundations* (London: Routledge and Kegan Paul, 1989), p. 106.
50. Ibid., p. 107.
51. These stages are described in detail in Rinpochay and Hopkins, *Death, Intermediate State and Rebirth*, pp. 13–20, 29–48.
52. Varela, *Sleeping, Dreaming, and Dying*, p. 125.
53. Padmasambhava, *Natural Liberation*, pp. 208–9.
54. Rinbochay and Hopkins, *Death, Intermediate State and Rebirth*, pp. 47–48.
55. Padmasambhava, *Natural Liberation*, p. 243.
56. Ibid., pp. 257–73.
57. See, for example, *The Life of Shabkar: The Autobiography of a Tibetan Yogin*, trans. Mattieu Ricard (Albany, NY: State University of New York Press, 1994), p. 94.
58. *Paṭṭhāna* I.312–13. Harvey, *The Selfless Mind*, p. 98.
59. Ibid., p. 99.
60. Ibid. According to Harvey, the *Kathāvathu* mentions the opposing view that all the sense organs are present from the beginning. There is no mention of implantation in the early accounts.

Chapter 8: The Ethical Urgency of Death

1. Geshey Ngawang Dhargyey, *Tibetan Tradition of Mental Development* (Dharamsala: Library of Tibetan Works & Archives, 1974), pp. 87–88.
2. Karma Lekshe Tsomo, *Sisters in Solitude: Two Traditions of Buddhist Monastic Ethics for Women, A Comparative Analysis of the Dharmagupta and Mūlasarvāstivāda Bhikṣuṇī Prātimokṣa Sūtras* (Albany, NY: State University of New York Press, 1996), p. 81.
3. Martin G. Wiltshire, "The 'Suicide' Problem in the Pāli Canon," in *Journal of International Association of Buddhist Studies* 6, 2 (1983): 124–40.
4. The *Fanwangjing* (*Brahmajala-sūtra*), source of the Chinese lineage of *bodhisattva* precepts, is not the same as the Indian text by the same name. The *Shoulangyanjing* (*Śūraṃgama-sūtra*) was also apparently composed in China. Jan Yün-hua [Ran Yunhua], "Buddhist Self-immolation in Medieval China," *History of Religions* 4 (1964–65): 243.
5. Ibid., p. 257.

6. Ibid., p. 246.

7. Ibid., p. 297.

8. Ibid., p. 299.

9. Kathryn Ann Tsai, trans., *Lives of the Nuns: Biographies of Buddhist Nuns from the Fourth to Sixth Centuries* (Honolulu: University of Hawaii Press, 1994), p. 60.

10. Ibid., pp. 79–80.

11. Ibid., pp. 80–81.

12. World Tibet Network News, April 29, 1998. (http://www.tibet.ca/wtnarchive/1998/4/29_5.html, 30_3.html)

13. Sallie B. King, "They Who Burn Themselves for Peace: Buddhist Self-Immolation," *Socially Engaged Buddhism for the New Millennium* (Bangkok: Sathirakoses-Nagapridipa Foundation and Foundation for Children, 1999), p. 392.

14. Ibid., p. 283.

15. Ibid., p. 284.

16. Ibid., p. 285.

17. Ibid., p. 59.

18. Cf., Judith Jarvis Thomson, "The Trolley Problem," in *Rights, Restitution, and Risk: Essays in Moral Theory* (Cambridge, MA: Harvard University Press, 1986), pp. 94–116.

19. Mark Tatz, trans., *The Skill in Means Sūtra (Upāya-kauśalya Sūtra)* (Delhi: Motilal Banarsidass, 1994), pp. 73–74.

20. King, "They Who Burn Themselves for Peace," p. 292.

21. Frances Kissling, *How to Talk about Abortion* (Washington, DC: Catholics for a Free Choice, 2000), pp. 10–11.

22. Somdetch Phra Mahā Samaṇa Chao Krom Phrayā Vajirañāṇavarorasa, *The Entrance to the Vinaya: Vinayamukha*, vol. 1 (Bangkok: Mahāmakuṭarājavidyālaya, 1969), p. 45.

23. The *daśakuśala* are to refrain from (1) killing, (2) stealing, (3) adultery, (4) lying, (5) divisive speech, (6) harsh speech, (7) idle gossip, (8) covetousness, (9) malice, and (10) wrong views.

24. Tsomo, *Sisters in Solitude*, pp. 46, 105.

25. Vajirañāṇvarorasa, *Entrance to the Vinaya*, p. 47.

26. Quoted by Buddhaghoṣa, *Path of Purification*, p. 249.

27. The four types of birth are: (1) from a womb, (2) from an egg, (3) from moisture, and (4) by apparition (*upapāduka*). Vasubandhu, *Abhidharmakośabhāṣyam*, pp. 380–81.

28. Damien Keown, *Buddhism and Bioethics* (New York: St. Martin's Press, 1995), p. 10.

29. Tenzin Gyatso, *Buddha Śākyamuni's Advice*, trans. Karma Lekshe Tsomo, unpublished manuscript, p. xiv.

30. Donden, *Health Through Balance*, p. 178.

31. These six conditions are: (1) the mother is ripe for conception; (2) the *bardo* being is present; (3) the parents engage in sexual intercourse; (4) the mother's womb is not defective; (5) the semen is not defective; and (6) the *bardo* being has created the causes to be born to these parents.

32. Rinpochay and Hopkins, *Death, Intermediate State and Rebirth*, p. 59.

33. Cait Collins, "Conception and the Entry of Consciousness: When Does a Life Begin?" in *Buddhist Women Across Cultures: Realizations*, ed. Karma Lekshe Tsomo (Albany, NY: State University of New York Press, 1999), pp. 197–98. The developmental stages of the fetus are described in Rinpochay and Hopkins, *Death, Intermediate State and Rebirth*, pp. 61–68; and in Rechung Rinpoche, *Tibetan Medicine* (Berkeley, CA: University of California Press, 1976), pp. 32–37.

34. For example, William R. LaFleur, *Liquid Life: Abortion and Buddhism in Japan* (Princeton, NJ: Princeton University Press, 1992).

35. Helen Hardacre, *Marketing the Menacing Fetus in Japan* (Berkeley, CA: University of California Press, 1997).

36. William R. LaFleur, "Contestation and Consensus: The Morality of Abortion in Japan," *Philosophy East and West* 40 (1990): 535.

37. Ibid.

38. Robert Aitken, *The Mind of Clover: Essays in Zen Buddhist Ethics* (San Francisco: North Point Press, 1984).

39. Yvonne Rand, "Abortion: A Respectful Meeting Ground," in *Buddhism Through American Women's Eyes*, ed. Karma Lekshe Tsomo (Ithaca, NY: Snow Lion Publications, 1995).

40. These ideas are framed in response to the Judith Jarvis Thomson's chapter, "A Defense of Abortion," in *Rights, Restitution, and Risk: Essays in Moral Theory* (Cambridge, MA: Harvard University Press, 1986), pp. 1–19.

41. In the Mahāyāna literature, the ten perfections are generosity (*dana*), ethical conduct (*śīla*), patience (*kṣānti*), joyful effort (*vīrya*), meditation (*dhyāna*), wisdom (*prājña*), skillful means (*upāya-kauśalya*), aspiration (*praṇidhāna*), power (*bala*), and exalted wisdom (*jñāna*). In the Pāli literature, they are generosity (*dana*), ethical conduct (*sila*), renunciation (*nekkhamma*), wisdom (*pañña*), energy (*viriya*), patience (*khanti*), truthfulness (*sacca*), determination (*aditthana*), loving kindness (*metta*), and equanimity (*upekkha*).

42. Thubten Zopa Rinpoche, *Chöd: Cutting Off the Truly-Existent "I"* (London: Wisdom Publications, 1983), p. 31.

43. See Margaret Coberly, *Sacred Passage: How to Provide Fearless, Compassionate Care for the Dying* (Boston: Shambhala, 2003).

Chapter 9: Extending Life and Hastening Death

1. Some have attempted to extend the meaning of *en* to "gentle" or "beautiful," but these are not accurate renderings of the Greek. Tom L. Beauchamp, *Intending Death: the Ethics of Assisted Suicide and Euthanasia* (Upper Saddle River, NJ: Prentice Hall, 1996), p. 2.

2. Katherine K. Young, "Euthanasia: Traditional Hindu Views and the Contemporary Debate," in *Hindu Ethics: Purity, Abortion, and Euthanasia*, ed. Harold G. Coward, Julius J. Lipner, and Katherine K. Young (Delhi: Sri Satguru Pulications, 1989), pp. 71–72.

3. Beauchamp, *Intending Death*, pp. 2–3.

4. Ibid., p. 3.

5. Alternatively, Ronald P. Hamel defines involuntary euthanasia as being achieved against the will of the patient and nonvoluntary euthanasia as being achieved without the consent of the patient. *Choosing Death: Active Euthanasia, Religion, and the Public Debate* (Philadelphia, PA: Trinity Press International, 1991), p. 43.

6. Tom L. Beauchamp, ed., *Intending Death: The Ethics of Assisted Suicide and Euthanasia* (Upper Saddle River, NJ: Prentice Hall, 1996), p. 4.

7. Young, "Euthanasia," p. 72.

8. Hamel, *Choosing Death*, p. 38.

9. Beauchamp, *Intending Death: the Ethics of Assisted Suicide and Euthanasia* (Upper Saddle River, NJ: Prentice Hall, 1996), p. 5.

10. Ibid., p. 149.

11. The popular myth that lemmings commit suicide has been rebutted by British naturalists who claim that, on the contrary, lemmings "have a well-honed instinct for survival." (http://www.affinity-systems.ab.ca/muse1/1042.html). In 1998, it was reported that a group of pilot whales had committed suicide in Tasmania; in fact, the whales had "determined to stay with a family group at the cost of their lives." (http://www.smh.com.au/news/9810/20/text/national7.html)

12. Keown, *Buddhism and Bioethics*, pp. 62–63.

13. See Buddhaghoṣa, *The Path of Purification*, p. 409; and Harvey, *The Selfless Mind*, p. 173.

14. Bhikkhu Thanissaro, *The Buddhist Monastic Code* (Valley Center, CA: Metta Forest Monastery, 1994), p. 70.

15. Beauchamp, *Intending Death*, pp. 5–11.

16. David Heyd, "The Meaning of Life and the Right to Voluntary Euthanasia," *Euthanasia*, ed. Amnon Carmi (Berlin: Springer-Verlag, 1984), pp. 169–73.

17. Ibid., p. 169.

18. Ibid., p. 171.

19. Ibid., p. 173.

20. Beauchamp, *Intending Death*, p. 7.

21. For example, see Gyalwa Gendun Druppa [First Dalai Lama], *Training the Mind in the Great Way*, trans. Glenn Mullin (Ithaca, NY: Snow Lion Publications, 1993).

22. Edmund D. Pellegrino, "The Place of Intention in the Moral Assessment of Assisted Suicide and Active Euthanasia," in *Intending Death*, p. 163.

23. Ibid. The same elements presumably apply to an immoral event.

24. Vasubhandu, *Abhidharmakośabhāṣyam*, p. 686.

25. This discussion draws on Hamel, *Choosing Death*, pp. 23–25, 36–43.

26. Personal communication with Margaret Coberly, R.N., August 8, 2000.

27. Keown, *Buddhism and Bioethics*, p. 156.

28. Beauchamp, *Intending Death*, p. 8.

29. Damien Keown, "Killing, Karma, and Caring: Euthanasia in Buddhism and Christianity, *Journal of Medical Ethics* 21:5 (1995): 265.

Chapter 10: Buddhism and Genetic Engineering

1. For an understanding of conception and embryology from a medical perspective, I gratefully acknowledge the comments of Dr. Yvonne Vaucher, professor of neonatologist at the University of California at San Dieco Medical Center, and Dr. Cynthia Geppert, assistant professor of Psychiatry and associate director of the Religious Studies Program at the University of New Mexico. All errors are my own.

2. The National Bioethics Advisory Commission report, *Ethical Issues in Human Stem Cell Research,* vol. 3, *Religious Perspectives,* June 2000, is available online: http://bioethics.gov/pubs.html#index.

3. Thomas A. Shannon and Allan B. Wolter, O. F. M., "Reflections on the Moral Status of the Preembryo," in *The New Genetic Medicine: Theological and Ethical Reflections,* eds. Thomas A. Shannon and James J. Walter (Lanham, MD: Rowman & Littlefield, 2003), p. 51.

4. Evelyn Falls, Joy Skeel, and Walter Edinger, "The Koan of Cloning: A Buddhist Perspective on the Ethics of Human Cloning Technology," (also subtitled, "Buddhism Challenges Western Notions of Identity, Altering the Terrain of the Cloning Debate"), *Second Opinion* (September 1999): 51.

5. Falls, Skeel, and Edinger, "The Koan of Cloning," p. 53. The article concludes with some highly debatable arguments about antilogic and the Absolute that undermine the ethical frame constructed earlier in the article.

6. On this point, see Erik Parens, "On the Ethics and Politics of Embryonic Stem Cell Research," Thomas A. Shannon, "From the Micro to the Macro," and Cynthia B. Cohen, "Leaps and Boundaries: Expanding Oversight of Human Stem Cell Research," in *The Human Embryonic Stem Cell Debate: Science, Ethics, and Public Policy,* eds. Suzanne Holland, Karen Lebacqz, and Laurie Zoloth (Cambridge and London: Massachusetts Institute of Technology Press, 2001), pp. 46–47, 177–78, and 212–14.

7. A synopsis of this history is found in Shannon and Wolter, *The New Genetic Medicine,* pp. 50–59.

8. John C. Fletcher, "NBAC [National Bioethiss Advisory Commission]'s Arguments on Embryo Research: Strengths and Weaknesses," in Holland, et al., *The Human Embryonic Stem Cell Debate,* pp. 61–72.

9. Susan Holland, "Beyond the Embryo: A Feminist Appraisal of the Embryonic Stem Cell Debate," *The Human Embryonic Stem Cell Debate,* pp. 73–86.

Bibliography

Aitken, Robert. *The Mind of Clover: Essays in Zen Buddhist Ethics*. San Francisco: North Point Press, 1984.

Anacker, Stefan, trans., and ed. *Seven Works of Vasubandhu: The Buddhist Psychological Doctor*. Delhi: Motilal Banarsidass, 1984.

Bansal, B. L. *Bön: Its Encounter with Buddhism in Tibet*. Delhi: Eastern Book Linkers, 1994.

Barua, Amala. *Mind and Mental Factors in Early Buddhist Psychology*. New Delhi: Northern Book Centre, 1990.

Battin, Margaret Pabst and D. J. Mayo, eds. *Suicide: The Philosophical Issues*. New York: St. Martin's Press, 1980.

Beauchamp, Tom L., and Robert Veatch, eds. *Ethical Issues in Death and Dying*. Englewood Cliffs, NJ: Prentice-Hall, 1996.

Beauchamp, Tom L. *Intending Death: the Ethics of Assisted Suicide and Euthanasia*. Upper Saddle River, NJ: Prentice-Hall, 1996.

Beauchamp, Tom L., and James F. Childress. *Principles of Biomedical Ethics*. New York: Oxford University Press, 1989.

Becker, Carl. *Breaking the Circle: Death and the Afterlife in Buddhism*. Carbondale, IL: Southern Illinois University Press, 1993.

———. "Buddhist Views of Suicide and Euthanasia." *Philosophy East and West* 40, No. 4 (1990): 543–54.

Benn, James A. "Where Text Meets Flesh: Burning the Body as an Apocryphal Practice in Chinese Buddhism." *History of Religions* 37, No. 4 (1998): 295–322.

Benson, Herbert, Robert A. F. Thurman, Howard E. Gardner, Daniel Goleman, eds. *MindScience: An East-West Dialogue*. Boston, MA: Wisdom Publications, 1991.

Brock, Dan. W. *Life and Death: Philosophical Essays in Biomedical Ethics.* New York: Cambridge University Press, 1993.

Brody, Baruch A. *Suicide and Euthanasia: Historical and Contemporary Themes.* Boston: Kluwer, 1989.

Brown, Brian Edward. *The Buddha Nature: A Study of the Tathāgatagarbha and Ālayavijñāna.* Delhi: Motilal Banarsidass Publishers, 1991.

Buddhaghoṣa, Bhadantācariya. *The Path of Purification (Visuddhimagga).* Translated by Bhikkhu Ñyāṇamoli. Colombo: A. Semage, 1964.

Burford, Grace G. *Desire, Death and Goodness: The Conflict of Ultimate Values in Theravāda Buddhism.* New York: Peter Lang, 1991.

Campbell, June. *Traveler in Space: In Search of Female Identity in Tibetan Buddhism.* New York: George Braziller, 1996.

Camus, Albert. *The Myth of Sisyphus and Other Essays.* Translated by Justin O'Brien. New York: Alfred A. Knopf, 1955.

———. *A Happy Death.* New York: Vintage Books, 1972.

Carrither, Michael, Steven Collins, and Steven Lukes, eds. *The Category of the Person: Anthropology, Philosophy, History.* Cambridge: Cambridge University Press, 1985.

Chakrabarti, Arindam. "But, Is Death an Evil?" and "Notes on Immortality." In *Sofies Welt: Ein interreligiöser Dialog über Geschichte, Philosophie und Wirklichkeit.* Rehbug-Loccum: Evangelische Akademie Loccum, 1998.

Chappell, David W., and Karma Lekshe Tsomo, eds. *Living and Dying in Buddhist Cultures.* Honolulu: University of Hawai'i Buddhist Studies Program, 1998.

Coberly, Margaret. *Sacred Passage: How to Provide Fearless, Compassionate Care for the Dying.* Boston: Shambhala, 2003.

Coberly, Margaret and S. I. Shapiro. "A Transpersonal Approach to Care of the Dying." *Journal of Transpersonal Psychology* 30, No. 1 (1998): 1–37.

Collins, Steven. *Selfless Persons: Imagery and Thought in Theravāda Buddhism.* Cambridge: Cambridge University Press, 1982.

Collins, Cait. "Conception and the Entry of Consciousness: When Does a Life Begin?" In *Buddhist Women Across Cultures: Realizations.* Edited by Karma Lekshe Tsomo. Albany, NY: State University of New York Press, 1999.

Conze, Edward, trans. *The Wisdom Books.* London: George Allen & Unwin, 1958.

Cozort, Daniel and Craig Preston. *Buddhist Philosophy: Losang Gönchok's Short Commentary to Jamyang Shayba's Root Text on Tenets.* Ithaca, NY: Snow Lion Publications, 2003.

Crawford, S. Cromwell. *Dilemmas of Life and Death: Hindu Ethics in a North American Context.* Delhi: Sri Satguru Publications, 1997.

Crick, Francis. *The Astonishing Hypothesis: The Scientific Search for the Soul.* New York: Scribner: Maxwell Macmillan International, 1994.

Cuevas, Bryan J. "Speculations on the Development of the Intermediate-State Doctrine in Tibet." Monograph presented at the XIIth Conference of the International Association of Buddhist Studies, Lausanne, August, 1999.

Davids-Rhys, T. W. and Hermann Oldenberg, trans. *Vinaya Texts.* Delhi: Motilal Banarsidass, 1982.

Davids-Rhys, T. W. and C. A. F. Rhys-Davids, trans. *Dialogue of the Buddha.* London: Pali Text Society, 1899–1921.

Dhargyey, Geshey Ngawang. *Tibetan Tradition of Mental Development.* Dharamsala: Library of Tibetan Works & Archives, 1974.

Donden, Yeshi. *Health Through Balance: An Introduction to Tibetan Medicine.* Ithaca, NY: Snow Lion Publications, 1986.

Drapper, Gyalwa Gendun. *Training the Mind in the Great Way.* Translated by Glen Mullin. Ithaca, NY: Snow Lion Publications, 1993.

Dworkin, Ronald. *Life's Dominion: An Argument about Abortion, Euthanasia, and Individual Freedom.* New York: Alfred A. Knopf, 1993.

Easwaran, Eknath, trans. *The Dhammapada.* Petaluma, CA: Nilgiri Press, 1985.

Eliade, Mircea. *Death, Afterlife and Eschatology: From Primitives to Zen: A Thematic Sourcebook of the History of Religions.* New York: Harper & Row, 1967.

Evans-Wentz, W. Y. *The Tibetan Book of the Dead.* London: Oxford University Press, 1960.

Falls, Evelyn, Joy Skeel, and Walter Edinger. "The Koan of Cloning: A Buddhist Perspective on the Ethics of Human Cloning Technology." *Second Opinion* (September, 1999).

Faure, Bernard. "The Ritualization of Death." *The Rhetoric of Immediacy: A Cultural Critique of Chan/Zen Buddhism.* Princeton, NJ: Princeton University Press, 1991.

Foot, Philippa. *Abortion: Moral and Legal Perspectives.* Edited by Jay L. Garfield and Patricia Hennessey. Amherst, MA: University of Massachusetts Press, 1984.

Fremantle, Francesca and Chögyam Trungpa. *The Tibetan Book of the Dead: The Great Liberation Through Hearing in the Bardo.* Boston: Shambhala, 1987.

Freud, Sigmund. *Civilization and Its Discontents.* Translated by James Strachey. New York: W. W. Norton and Co., 1962.

Friedman, Maurice. "Death and the Dialogue with the Absurd." *The Phenomenon of Death: Faces of Mortality.* Edited by Edith Wyschogrod. New York: Harper & Row, 1973.

Gervais, Karen Grandstrand. *Redefining Death.* New Haven, CT: Yale University Press, 1986.

Gómez, Luis O. *Land of Bliss: The Paradise of the Buddha of Measureless Light: Sanskrit and Chinese Versions of the Sukhāvatīvyūha Sūtras.* Honolulu: University of Hawai'i Press, 1996.

Griffiths, Paul J. *On Being Mindless: Buddhist Meditation and the Mind-Body Problem.* La Salle, IL: Open Court, 1986.

Guenther, Herbert V. *The Life and Teaching of Nāropa.* Boston and London: Shambhala, 1986.

Guenther, Herbert V. and Leslie S. Kawamura. *Mind in Buddhist Psychology* Emeryville, CA: Dharma Publishing, 1975.

Gyatso, Janet. "The Gcod Tradition." In *Soundings in Tibetan Civilization.* Edited by Barbara Nimmri Aziz and Matthew Kapstein. New Delhi: Manohar, 1985.

Hamada, Harold Tooru. *The Role of Death in Buddhist Thought*. Master's thesis, University of Hawai'i, 1968.

Hamel, Ronald P. *Choosing Death: Active Euthanasia, Religion, and the Public Debate*. Philadelphia: Trinity Press International, 1991.

Hardacre, Helen. *Marketing the Menacing Fetus in Japan*. Berkeley, CA: University of California Press, 1997.

Harrison, Paul. "Who Gets to Ride in the Great Vehicle? Self-Image and Identity Among the Followers of the Early Mahāyāna." *Journal of the International Association of Buddhist Studies* 10 (1987): 67–89.

Harvey, Peter. *The Selfless Mind: Personality, Consciousness, and Nirvāṇa in Early Buddhism*. Surrey, England: Curzon Press, 1995.

Hayes, Richard P. *Dignāga on the Interpretation of Signs*. Dordrect: Kluwer, 1988.

Hayward, Jeremy. *Shifting Worlds, Changing Minds: Where the Sciences and Buddhism Meet*. Boston: Shambala Publications, 1987.

Heyd, David. "The Meaning of Life and the Right to Voluntary Euthanasia." In *Euthanasia*. Edited by Amnon Carmi. Berlin: Springer-Verlag, 1984.

Hirabayashi, Jay and Shotaro Iida. "Another Look at the Mādhyamika vs. Yogācāra Controversy Concerning Existence and Non-Existence." *Prajñāpāramitā and Related Systems*. Edited by Lewis Lancaster. Berkeley, CA: University of California Buddhist Studies Series, 1977.

Holk, Fredrick H., ed. *Death and Eastern Thought: Understanding Death in Eastern Religions and Philosophies*. Nashville, TN: Abingdon Press, 1974.

Holland, Suzanne, Karen Lebacqz, and Laurie Zoloth, eds. *The Human Embryonic Stem Cell Debate: Science, Ethics, and Public Policy*. Cambridge and London: Massachusetts Institute of Technology Press, 2001.

Hopkins, Jeffrey. "Death, Sleep, and Orgasm: Gateways to the Mind of Clear Light." *Living and Dying in Buddhist Cultures*. Edited by David W. Chappell and Karma Lekshe Tsomo. Honolulu: Univerity of Hawai'i Buddhist Studies Program, 1998.

———. *Meditations of Emptiness*. London: Wisdom Publications, 1983.

———. *Buddhist Advice for Living and Liberation: Nāgārjuna's Precious Garland*. Ithaca, NY: Snow Lion Publications, 1998.

Houshmand, Zara, Robert B. Livingston, and B. Alan Wallace. *Consciousness at the Crossroads: Conversations with the Dalai Lama on Brain Science and Buddhism*. Ithaca, NY: Snow Lion Publications, 1991.

———. "A Tibetan Perspective on the Nature of Spiritual Experience." In *Paths to Liberation: The Mārga and Its Transformations in Buddhist Thought*. Edited by Robert E. Buswell Jr., and Robert M. Gimello. Honolulu: University of Hawaii Press, 1992.

Humphry, Derek. *Dying with Dignity: Understanding Euthanasia*. Secaucus, NJ: Carol Publishing Group, 1992.

Humphry, Derek and Ann Wickett. *The Right to Die: Understanding Euthanasia*. New York: Harper and Row, 1986.

Iida, Shotam. "The Nature of Saṃvṛti and the Relationship of Paramārtha to It In Svātantrika-Mādhyamika." In *The Problem of Two Truths in Bud-*

dhism and Vedānta. Edited by Mervyn Sprung. Dordrecht: D. Reidel Publishing Company, 1973.

Jan Yün-hua. "Buddhist Self-immolation in Medieval China." *History of Religions* 4 (1964–65): 243–68.

Kapleau, Philip. *The Wheel of Life and Death.* New York: Doubleday, 1989.

Kastenbaum, Robert J. *Death, Society, and Human Experience.* St. Louis: C. V. Mosby, 1981.

Katherine K. Young, "Euthanasia: Traditional Hindu Views and the Contemporary Debate." *Hindu Ethics: Purity, Abortion, and Euthanasia.* Edited by Harold G. Coward, Julius J. Lipner, and Katherine K. Young. Delhi: Sri Satguru Publications, 1989.

Keown, Damien. *The Nature of Buddhist Ethics.* New York: St. Martin's Press, 1992.

———. "Karma, Character, and Consequentialism." *Journal of Religious Ethics* 24, No. 2 (1996): 329–49.

———. *Buddhism and Bioethics.* New York: St. Martin's Press, 1995.

———. ed. *Buddhism and Abortion.* Honolulu: University of Hawaii Press, 1999.

———. "Killing, Karma and Caring: Euthanasia in Buddhism and Christianity." *Journal of Medical Ethics* 21, No. 5 (1995): 265.

King, Sallie B. King. "They Who Burn Themselves for Peace: Buddhist Self-Immolation." In *Socially Engaged Buddhism for the New Millennium.* Bangkok: Sathirakoses-Nagapridipa Foundation & Foundation for Children, 1999.

Kirk, G. S. and J. E. Raven, trans. *The Pre-Socratic Philosophers: A Critical History.* Cambridge: Cambridge University Press, 1957.

Kissling, Frances. *How to Talk about Abortion.* Washington, DC: Catholics for a Free Choice, 2000.

Klein, Anne Carolyn. *Knowledge and Liberation.* Ithaca, NY: Snow Lion Publications, 1986.

———. *Naming, Knowing and Negation.* Ithaca, NY: Snow Lion Publications, 1991.

Kleinig, John. *Valuing Life.* Princeton, NJ: Princeton University Press, 1991.

Kuhse, Helga. "Euthanasia." *A Companion to Ethics.* Edited by Peter Singer. Cambridge: Blackwell, 1991.

LaFleur, William R. "Contestation and Consensus: The Morality of Abortion in Japan." *Philosophy East and West* 40 (1990): 529–42.

———. *Liquid Life: Abortion and Buddhism in Japan.* Princeton, NJ: Princeton University Press, 1992.

Lauf, Detlef Ingo. *Secret Doctrines of the Tibetan Books of the Dead.* Translated by Graham Parkes. Boston: Shambhala, 1977.

Lecso, Phillip A. "Euthanasia: A Buddhist Perspective." *Journal of Religion and Health* 25, No. 1 (1986): 51–57.

Levine, George, ed. *Constructions of the Self.* New Brunswick, NJ: Rutgers University Press, 1992.

Lipner, Julius J. "The Classical Hindu View on Abortion and the Moral Status of the Unborn." In *Hindu Ethics: Purity, Abortion, and Euthanasia.* Edited by Harold G. Coward, Julius J. Lipner, and Kathering K. Young. Delhi: Sri Satguru Publications, 1989.

Loden, Geshe Acharya Thubten. *The Fundamental Potential for Enlightenment.* Melbourne: Tushita Publications, 1996.

Lodö, Lama. *Bardo Teachings: The Way of Death and Rebirth.* San Francisco: KDK Publications, 1982.

Lopez, Donald S. " 'Lamaism' and the Disappearance of Tibet." In *Constructing Tibetan Culture: Contemporary Perspectives.* Edited by Frank J. Korom. Quebec: World Heritage Press, 1997.

Loy, David. "The Nonduality of Life and Death: A Buddhist View of Repression." *Philosophy East and West* 40, No. 2 (1990): 151–74.

Markus, Hazel Rose and Shinobu Kitayama. "The Cultural Construction of Self and Emotion: Implications of Social Behavior. In *Emotion and Culture: Empirical Studies of Mutual Influence.* Edited by Shinobu Kitayama and Hazel Rose Markus. Washington, DC: American Psychological Association, 1994.

Matthews, Bruce. "Post-Classical Developments in the Concepts of Karma and Rebirth in Theravāda Buddhism." In *Karma and Rebirth: Post Classical Developments.* Edited by Ronald W. Neufeldt. Albany, NY: State University of New York Press, 1986.

McDermott, James P. "Karma and Rebirth in Early Buddhism." *Karma and Rebirth in Classical Indian Traditions.* Edited by Wendy Doniger O'Flaherty. Berkeley, CA: University of California Press, 1980.

Ming-Wood, Liu. "The Yogācāra and Mādhyamika Interpretations of the Buddha-nature Concept of Chinese Buddhism. *Philosophy East and West* 35, 2 (1985): 171–93.

Mullin, Glenn H., trans. and ed. *Living in the Face of Death: The Tibetan Tradition.* Ithaca, NY: Snow Lion Publications, 1998.

Murcott, Susan. *The First Buddhist Women: Translations and Commentaries on the Therigatha.* Berkeley, CA: Parallax Press, 1991.

Nagao, Gadjin M. *Mādhyamika and Yogācāra: A Study of Mahāyāna Philosophies.* Albany, NY: State University of New York Press, 1991.

Nagel, Thomas. *Mortal Questions.* Cambridge University Press, 1979.

Napper, Elizabeth. *Dependent-Arising and Emptiness.* Boston: Wisdom Publications, 1989.

Neufeldt, Ronald W., ed. *Karma and Rebirth: Post Classical Developments.* Albany, NY: State University of New York Press, 1986.

Neumaier-Dargyay, Eva K. "Buddhism." In *Life after Death in World Religions.* Edited by Harold Coward. Delhi: Sri Satguru Publications, 1997.

O'Flaherty, Wendy Doniger, ed. *Karma and Rebirth in Classical Indian Traditions.* Berkeley, CA: University of California, 1980.

Obayashi, Hiroshi, ed. *Death and Afterlife: Perspectives of World Religions.* New York: Greenwood Press, 1992.

Ohnuki-Tierney, Emiko. "Brain Death and Organ Transplantation: Cultural Bases of Medical Technology." *Current Anthropology* 35, No. 3 (1994): 233–54.

Orofino, Giacomella. *Sacred Tibetan Teachings on Death and Liberation: Texts from the Most Ancient Traditions of Tibet.* Dorset, England: Prism Press, 1990.

Padmasambhava. *Natural Liberation: Padmasambhava's Teachings on the Six Bardos.* Translated by B. Alan Wallace. Boston: Wisdom Publications, 1998.

———. *The Tibetan Book of Living and Dying.* Translated by Robert A. F. Thurman, New York: Bantam Books, 1994.

Parfit, Derek. "Personal Identity." *Philosophical Review* 80 (1971): 3–27.

Parkes, Graham. "Death and Detachment: Montaigne, Zen, Heidegger, and the Rest." *Death and Philosophy.* Edited by Jeff Malpas and Robert C. Solomon. London: Routledge and Kegan Paul, 1998.

Pellegrino, Edmund D. "The Place of Intention in the Moral Assessment of Assisted Suicide and Active Euthanasia." In *Intending Death: the Ethics of Assisted Suicide and Euthanasia.* Edited by Tom L. Beauchamp. Upper Saddle River, NJ: Prentice-Hall, 1996.

Perdue, Daniel E. *Debate in Tibetan Buddhism.* Ithaca, NY: Snow Lion Publications, 1992.

Perrett, Roy W. *Death and Immortality.* Dordrecht, Netherlands: Martinus Nijhoff Pulbishers, 1987.

Pesala, Bhikkhu. *The Debate of King Milinda.* Delhi: Motilal Banarsidass, 1998.

Powers, John. *Introduction to Tibetan Buddhism.* Ithaca, NY: Snow Lion Publications, 1995.

Quill, Timothy E. *Death and Dignity: Making Choices and Taking Charge.* New York: W. W. Norton & Co., 1993.

Rabten, Geshe. *The Mind and its Functions.* Le Mont-Pelerin, Switzerland: Editions Rabten Choeling, 1992.

Rachels, James. *The End of Life: Euthanasia and Morality.* Oxford: Oxford University Press, 1986.

Rand, Yvonne. "Abortion: A Respectful Meeting Ground." In *Buddhism Through American Women's Eyes.* Edited by Karma Lekshe Tsomo. Ithaca, NY: Snow Lion Publications, 1995.

Rangdrol, Tsele Natsok. *The Mirror of Mindfulness: The Cycle of the Four Bardos.* Boston: Shambhala, 1989.

Rawlinson, Andrew. "The Position of the *Aṣṭasāhasrikā Prajñāpāramitā* in the Development of Early Mahāyāna." *Prajñāpāramitā and Related Texts.* Berkeley, CA: University of California Buddhist Studies Series, 1977.

Raymond, Diane. "Fatal Practices: A Feminist Analysis of Physician-Assisted Suicide and Euthanasia." *Hypatia* 14 (Spring 1999): 1–25.

Regan, Tom, ed. *Matters of Life and Death: New Introductory Essays in Moral Philosophy.* New York: Random House, 1993.

Reynolds, Frank E. "Death as Threat, Death as Achievement: Buddhist Perspectives with Particular Reference to the Theravāda Tradition." *Death and Afterlife: Perspectives of World Religions.* Edited by Hiroshi Obayashi. New York: Greenwood Press, 1992.

Rinbochay, Lati and Elizabeth Napper. *Mind in Tibetan Buddhism.* Ithaca, NY: Snow Lion Publications, 1980.

Rinchen, Geshe Sonam. *Atiśa's Lamp for the Path to Enlightenment.* Translated and edited by Ruth Sonam. Ithaca, NY: Snow Lion Publications, 1997.

Rinpochay, Lati and Jeffrey Hopkins. *Death, Intermediate State and Rebirth in Tibetan Buddhism.* London: Rider and Company, 1979.

Rinpoche, Bokar. *Death and the Art of Dying in Tibetan Buddhism.* San Francisco, CA: Clear Point Press, 1993.

Rinpoche, Chökyi Nyima. *The Bardo Guidebook.* Hong Kong: Rangjung Yeshe, 1991.

Rinpoche, Rechung. *Tibetan Medicine.* Berkeley, CA: University of California Press, 1976.

Rinpoche, Sogyal. *The Tibetan Book of Living and Dying.* San Francisco, CA: Harper, 1992.

Rinpoche, Thubten Zopa. *Chöd: Cutting Off the Truly-Existent "I."* London: Wisdom Publications, 1983.

Samuel, Geoffrey. *Civilized Shamans: Buddhism in Tibetan Societies.* Washington, DC: Smithsonian Institution Press, 1993.

Sangay, Thupten. "Tibetan Ritual for the Dead." *Tibetan Medicine* 7 (1984): 30–40.

Schmithausen, Lambert. *Ālayavijñāna: On the Origin and the Early Development of a Central Concept of Yogācāra Philosophy,* Part I. Tokyo: International Institute for Buddhist Studies, 1987.

Schopen, Gregory. "The Suppression of Nuns and the Ritual Murder of their Special Dead in Two Buddhist Monastic Texts." *Journal of Indian Philosophy* 24 (1996): 563–92.

———. "An Old Inscription from Amarāvatī and the Cult of the Local Monastic Dead in Indian Buddhist Monasteries." *Journal of the International Association of Buddhist Studies* 14 (1991): 99–137.

———. "Ritual Rights and Bones of Contention: More on Monastic Funerals and Relics in the Mūlasarvāstivāda-vinaya." *Journal of Indian Philosophy* 22 (1994): 31–80.

Scott, G. E. *Moral Personhood: An Essay in the Philosophy of Moral Psychology.* Albany, NY: State University of New York Press, 1990.

Settar, S. *Pursuing Death: Philosophy and Practice of Voluntary Termination of Life.* Dharwad, Karnataka: Institute of Indian Art History, 1990.

Shannon, Thomas A., and James J. Walter. *The New Genetic Medicine: Theological and Ethical Reflections.* Lanham, MD: Rowman & Littlefield, 2003.

Sopa, Geshe Lhundup and Jeffrey Hopkins. *Practice and Theory of Tibetan Buddhism* Bombay: B. I. Publications, 1977.

Sparham, Gareth, trans. *Ocean of Eloquence: Tsong kha pa's Commentary of the Yogācāra Doctrine of Mind.* Albany, NY: State University of New York Press, 1993.

Stablein, William. "Medical Soteriology of Karma in Buddhist Tantra." In *Karma and Rebirth in Classical Indian Traditions.* Edited by Wendy Doniger O'Flaherty. Berkeley, CA: University of California Press, 1980.

Steinbock, Bonnie and Alastair Norcross. *Killing and Letting Die.* New York: Fordham University Press, 1994.

Tatz, Mark. *Asaṅgha's Chapter on Ethics: With the Commentary of Tsong-kha-pa.* Lewiston: Mellen Press, 1981.

———. trans. *The Skill in Means Sūtra (Upāya-kauśalya Sūtra).* Delhi: Motilal Banarsidass, 1994.

Taylor, Charles. *Sources of the Self.* Cambridge, MA: Harvard University Press, 1989.

Teiser, Stephen F. *Scripture on the Ten Kings and the Making of Purgatory in Medieval Chinese Buddhism.* Honolulu: University of Hawaii Press, 1994.

———. *Ghost Festivals in Medieval China.* Princeton, NJ: Princeton University Press, 1988.

Thanissaro, Bhikkhu. *The Buddhist Monastic Code.* Valley Center, CA: Metta Forest Monastery, 1994.

Thomson, Judith Jarvis. *Rights, Restitution, and Risk: Essays in Moral Theory.* Cambridge, MA: Harvard University Press, 1986.

Thurman, Robert A. F., trans. *The Tibetan Book of the Dead.* New York: Bantam Books, 1994.

Tsai, Kathryn Ann, trans. *Lives of the Nuns: Biographies of Buddhist Nuns From the Fourth to Sixth Centuries.* Honolulu: University of Hawaii Press, 1994.

Tsomo, Karma Lekshe. *Sisters in Solitude: Two Traditions of Buddhist Monastic Ethics for Women, A Comparative Analysis of the Dharmagupta and Mūlasarvāstivāda Bhikṣuṇī Prātimokṣa Sūtras.* Albany, NY: State University of New York Press, 1996.

———. "Organ Donation: Opportunity or Obstacle?" In *Tricycle* 11:4 (Summer 1993): 30–35.

Van Evra, James. "On Death as a Limit." *Language, Metaphysics, and Death.* Edited by John Donnelly. New York: Fordham University Press, 1978.

Varela, Francisco J. *Sleeping, Dreaming, and Dying: An Exploration of Consciousness with the Dalai Lama.* Boston: Wisdom Publications, 1997.

Vasubandhu. *Abhidharmakośabhāsyam.* Vol. II. Translated by Louis de La Vallée Poussin and Leo M. Pruden. Berkeley, CA: Asian Humanities Press, 1988.

———. *Vimsatukā-vijñāptimātratā-siddhi.* Translated by N. Aiyaswami Sastrin. Gangtok, Sikkim: Namgyal Institute of Tibetology, 1964.

Veatch, Robert M. *Death, Dying, and the Biological Revolution: Our Last Quest for Responsibility.* New Haven, CT: Yale University Press, 1989.

Vyanjana. *Theravāda Buddhist Ethics with Special Reference to Visuddhimagga.* Calcutta: Punthi Pustak, 1992.

Wallace, B. Alan. *Tibetan Buddhism from the Ground Up: A Practical Approach to Modern Life.* Boston: Wisdom Publications, 1993.

Wangyal, Tenzin. *Wonders of the Natural Mind: The Essence of Dzogchen in the Native Bön Tradition of Tibet.* Barrytown, NY: Station Hill Press, 1993.

Wayman, Alex. "The Intermediate-state Dispute in Buddhism." *Buddhist Studies in Honour of I. B. Horner.* Edited by L. Cousins, A. Kunst, and K. R. Norman. Dordrecht, Holland: D. Reidel, 1974.

Wicks, Robert. "The Therapeutic Psychology of *The Tibetan Book of the Dead.*" *Philosophy East and West* 47 (1997): 479–94.

Weir, Robert F. *Ethical Issues in Death and Dying*. New York: Columbia University Press, 1986.

Williams, Paul. *Mahāyāna Buddhism: The Doctrinal Foundations*. London: Routledge and Kegan Paul, 1989.

Willis, Janice Dean. *On Knowing Reality: The Tattvārtha Chapter of Asaṅga's Bodhisattvakhūmi*. New York: Columbia University Press, 1986.

Wilson, Joe. *Chandrakīrti's Sevenfold Reasoning: Meditation on the Selflessness of Persons*. Dharamsala: Library of Tibetan Works and Archives, 1980.

Wiltshire, Martin G. "The 'Suicide' Problem in the Pāli Canon." *Journal of International Association of Buddhist Studies* 6, No. 2 (1983): 124–40.

Young, Katherine K. "Euthanasia: Traditional Hindu Views and the Contemporary Debate." In *Hindu Ethics: Purity, Abortion, and Euthanasia*. Edited by Harold G. Coward, Julius J. Lipner, and Katherine K. Young. Delhi: Sri Satguru Publications, 1989.

Index